The GHG Method

A No Bullshit Approach To
Losing Body Fat, Upgrading Your Mind Set
& Radically Changing Your Life

Gav Gillibrand

DEDICATION

I'd like to dedicate this book to three special people in my life. My daughter Mia, aged 14, my baby boy Gabriel, aged 15 months, and my fiancée, soon to be wife, Alex. You guys are the reason I get up early and work hard at everything I do. You inspire me to be the best man I can be and keep me grounded when I get too big for my boots, which apparently, appears to be quite frequently. Thank you.

CONTENTS

ACKNOWLEDGMENTS

I'd like to thank quite a few people so please bear with me.
Firstly, I'd like to thank Mr. Tim Drummond. He was **my** coach and a brilliant one at that. He made me realise the power of effective coaching in this industry & true behavioural change. He also taught me to stop messing around and "grow a pair" and to move from a personal trainer in the city of London to an online fitness & nutrition coach with the ability to help clients all over the world. Thank you, sir.

Thanks must also go to Phil Hawksworth for helping and guiding me through the painful process of getting all I wanted to say onto paper and transforming my illegible mess into "something" that half resembles a book.

I'd like to thank Rachel Holmes for her book writing wisdom, her "motivational muses" and being a great friend.

I'd also like to say thanks to the following gentlemen. This is in no particular order:

Tony Robbins, Robin Sharma, Charles Poliquin, Gary Vaynerchuk, "The Rock", Joe Rogan, Wim Hof, David Goggins, Jim Kwik, Aubrey Marcus, Rob Moore, Eric Thomas, Jesse Itzler, Bedros Keulian, Lewis Howes, Ed Mylett, Craig Ballantyne, Ryan Holiday, Ben Greenfield, Jon Romaniello, Tim Ferris, John McAvoy, Rich Roll, James Clear, Shawn Stevenson, Paul Mort, Phil Learney, Ross Edgley & Jocko Willink.

Through their live events, books, emails, podcasts and social media posts, these guys have taught and inspired me on some level, either in person or from afar. The knowledge and wisdom bestowed has been graciously received, so thank you. They've also confirmed my belief that we, as humans, have so much untapped potential and that there is really no limit to what we can achieve in this life if we put our mind to it and really do the work. #GetShitDone

Thanks to my mum and dad because if they hadn't…

…well, you all know how that works don't you?

1. INTRODUCTION

"She picked that bloody stripper, Gavin from Kings Lynn. Not that I remember the details or anything".

Those were the words famous comedian Ed Byrne said with shock and an "I can't fucking believe it" attitude when asked about his first appearance on TV. "I was one of the few people that didn't get picked and it still hurts. It's still very raw".

That's right. I was chosen ahead of famous Dubliner, comedian Ed Byrne, on **the** programme to watch on a Saturday night in the late 80s and 90s: Blind Date. Hosted by the late, great Cilla Black, Blind Date was watched by up to 16 million people every Saturday night. Ed was funny as hell even then. Both the audience and Cilla were in stitches as he used his smooth Irish charm in an attempt to win over Sally from Bournemouth.

I will return to Blind Date very soon. First allow me to back up a little. At school, when they sent everyone out on work experience, rather than going the traditional route like most to an office, bank, or insurance company, I chose to go to the gym. My obsession with bodybuilding, mixed with the fact that Madonna (my future wife) at the time, had a good-looking, muscular personal trainer working out with her whenever she went running, was enough for me to decide that I wanted to be personal trainer to the stars. I want to clarify now that Madonna has never been, nor ever will be my wife; but at 14/15 years old, I dreamt it just might happen one day.

There I am, 9 o'clock Monday morning. It's 1989 and I've just arrived at the gym in Norwich for my first day of work experience. The owner, and retired bodybuilder Chris, is showing me around and then says, "let's have a workout". He sits me down on the leg press with 1x20kg plate per side and asks me to do 15 reps. No problem. The second I'd finished the set, he put on another plate each side. "15 reps, please".

Now I'm working a little, my legs are getting a good pump. Set finished. He adds another plate on each side. We now have 60kg on both sides for a total of 120kg. Not a huge weight in itself, but after 30 reps previously with very little rest, I have to dig deep to finish the set.

I manage to get the last few reps before slumping out. I'm sweating profusely, my legs are blown up and feeling like jelly, and my heart is pounding like a jackhammer. I know I've come to the right place. Out of the corner of my eye, I see a really good-looking guy. Tall, lean, tanned, with a ponytail, wearing a leotard. Yes, it's 1989 and step aerobics is the big new craze to hit the UK. I watch him take 30 or so women aged 25 to 55 through a workout to music on the steps, holding them all like warm putty in the palm of his hand. This is the point I say to myself, "that's who I want to be". Minus the ponytail. And the leotard. Although later in life, the leotard will play a role in another way. A different leotard, of course, not the one the step instructor was wearing.

In the year between A levels and going to university, I worked at a local sports centre in King's Lynn as a fitness instructor with the aim of getting some experience in the industry. "Experience", AKA: not getting the grades you need and having to wait a year before you can reapply for university. A few months into the job, I see it on the staff notice board. I don't know who put it there or why, but I'm glad they did. My eyes light up as I read out loud the words, "auditions for Blind Date".

Off I go to the Crown Hotel in Norwich for the first of three auditions. I find myself in a room full of egotistical wannabes desperate to get on TV. Satisfied I'm in the correct room, I proceed to bullshit my way through the first audition by telling the girl asking the questions that I'm a stripper.

"What's your favourite costume and what was the most embarrassing thing ever to happen to you on a gig?" asked the interviewer from ITV. "Some girl pulled my G-string and it ripped. I'm left naked in the middle of the pub", I lied. "Oh my god, what did you do?" she enquired. "What anyone would do, given the circumstances. I covered both my nipples and walked off the stage", winking at the interviewer. "That ought to do it", I whisper to myself.

I was quite pleased with how the bullshit flowed to be honest. In fairness, this wasn't a complete lie. Literally just a few weeks previously I'd auditioned after seeing an advert for "Strippograms Wanted" in the local paper. For those unfamiliar with the term, a strippogram involves appearing at an event such as a birthday party, hen do, or something similar, dressed in a costume with the view to taking your clothes off as a special surprise to the unsuspecting birthday girl or hen, in exchange for a stack of cash. I was offered the job and ended up doing my first gig a few weeks later at a pub in Cambridge dressed as a policeman. Getting semi-naked dancing to Michael Jackson's "Billie Jean" pumping out of my portable ghetto blaster. It's 1993 and yes, the ghetto blaster is still cool (ish).

Back to ITV Studios on the South Bank and Blind Date. Sitting to my left is a Scotsman with the broadest Glaswegian accent I've ever heard and, on my right, a funny, smooth-talking Irish man with all the charm of your favourite leprechaun.

"Here's a little poem from your favourite Dubliner Ed, I'm not feeling myself tonight so do you mind if I feel you instead". The crowd erupts with laughter. Sally is in stitches and Cilla nearly wets herself. Ed's opening gambit had scored big time with everyone in the studio, so I'm going to have to go all in to pull this one off. I don't remember exactly what I said, but I know it included the words "Adonis, truncheon, and naked". It appears to do the trick, as much to mine and Ed's amazement, she picks me. I can see it clear as day even now: Ed's face visibly shocked that she went for me. In this case, Sally clearly preferred the thought of a hunky stripper on her arm to a charming Irishman with an accent as smooth as blackstrap molasses.

The screen went back and there stands Sally with Cilla. I'd always said to myself that if I got picked, I'll ask Cilla if I can pick the card, so I do. I pick one of the cards from the three and hand it back to Cilla. "A trip on a steam train to the Nene Valley railway in Peterborough".

"I live there, Cilla", I say. "What?" "I live about 40 minutes from there", with a mixture of sarcasm and disappointment.

At the time I'm living with my parents on RAF Marham, near King's Lynn in Norfolk. I thought they must have been winding me up. I've packed for a hot destination. Got my swim shorts, t-shirts, vests, flip-flops, even suncream, ready for a week in the Caribbean or somewhere equally exotic. When the letter arrived to say that I had made it onto the show, it said, "Please pack for both cold and hot destinations". I realised that if I were picked, we would be leaving the very next morning after the show. The crowd are screaming and laughing. Cilla is in stiches. Sally is visibly disappointed, as am I, to be honest. We hold hands, walk off, turning back to wave to the audience and TV cameras as instructed.

Chatting to Sally, she seems like a nice girl. That night, we're taken to Planet Hollywood for a fat juicy burger and chips, a few beers, and a chat about how the next day is going to go. The chap who was assigned to look after us, a Scouser whose name escapes me, asks us questions about what clothes we had with us to wear. I say, "I've got a pair of cut-off denim shorts I was hoping to wear abroad in a sunny country. Shall I just wear them anyway?"

His eyes light up, as he knew he had a winner here. I'm confident, arrogant even, and prepared to do anything to show off. Perfect fodder for TV. He must have been chuckling to himself all night. It was after midnight before Sally and I go to bed. In separate beds, for the moment, at least. We have an early cab to Battersea helipad in West London tomorrow. Yep, we are travelling in style to the Nene Valley Railway, due to land at a luxury hotel in just a few hours time.

Picture the scene if you will. It's a beautiful sunny morning with a splendid Georgian country manor house in the background. You can hear the whir of the helicopter blades as the camera pans up and meets a chopper about to land on the lawn of the hotel. You'd expect to see someone at least semi-famous ducking their head as they step out of the helicopter. Sally steps out, looking great. I'm next, wearing trainers, cut off denim shorts, a Nike sweatshirt with a tan cultivated from hours on the sunbed that would make David Dickinson proud.

"Welcome to the hotel", said the manager as he briskly shook our hands.

"So, what we need Gavin and Sally, is just some general chat and banter on the train. Sally, you could ask Gavin if he would like to stoke your fire, you know, something like that", the director chuckles, clearly amused by his own humour. The director, two cameramen, a guy holding a boom for sound, a girl with a clipboard, and a chap for lighting are all gathered around on the platform as the train stands stationary on the track, waiting to take Sally and I on a jolly little jaunt through the Cambridgeshire countryside.

"How about I take my top off so I'm just wearing my denim shorts?" As I said, perfect TV material. Prepared to make a complete dick of myself for free. I'm in nothing more than cut-off denim shorts (staple stripper costume) and a pair of trainers, doing press ups on the platform to pump up for the cameras, when miraculously a bottle of baby oil appears. I say miraculously, but it was planned to perfection. I'd brought some of my "kit" along with me on the off chance that I might need it. It was a calculated move that paid off handsomely, as within a few minutes I have Sally oiling me up and someone else spraying me with water for that glistening, "I've just stepped out of the gym hot, sweaty, and extremely sexy" look that you all know and probably hate. Pumped up and ready to rock, I think to myself, "this is it, I will probably be famous after this". TV, magazines, and even Hollywood calling. OK, Hollywood was a stretch, but I really thought this could be my big break.

I'm on the train with the driver's cap on, bare chest pumped up and "sweating"; shovelling coal into the train's engine as Sally is tooting the horn. Casey Jones eat your heart out. It brings a smile to my face when I think back to it now. The director and his crew loved it. I'd gone through all those auditions, three of them, served them up my best bullshit to get on the show (although by now I WAS stripping) and they send me to bloody Peterborough for a trip on a steam train. They'd stitched me up good and proper.

A week later, I'm back at ITV's studio on the South Bank to film what they call the "Mishmash". This means Sally and I are asked questions about what we think of each other, how the date went, and so on. This section is shown when you go back on the live show with Cilla. How it's supposed to work is that the interviewer asks a question and I have to answer, while including the question in the answer, so the viewer can understand the context.

"Tell me about Sally's tattoo, Gav, and the fact she likes a drink and a cigarette". I think Sally had smoked a few cigarettes and enjoyed a pint on the date. He's goading me. Telling me she'd said some stuff about me that was "pretty cutting", I take the bait hook, line, and sinker. What a sucker. The bastard.

"She's got a huge tattoo on her arm, she drinks like a fish and smokes like a chimney, she's more of a bloke than I am… but don't put that bit in, I can't say that about her, can I? It's a bit too much I think".

Back on the South bank at ITV's studio. It's Saturday night and the follow-up is due to be filmed. I'm quite excited and a little nervous to see what Sally has said about me. I said a few cheeky remarks about Sally but asked them not to be shown. They wouldn't stitch me up again, would they?

"The screen went back and instead of seeing a tall, bronzed Adonis, I saw a short, stocky midget in cowboy boots", said Sally. The videotape continues to play. I'm sat on the sofa in front of a live audience of about 500 people. "I didn't fancy Gav in the slightest, Cilla". I try to speak but nothing comes out of my mouth. I'm lost for words for the first and only time in my life.

"Short, stocky midget in cowboy boots!" What?! "Respond Gav, quick. Before it's too late". My heart is racing, head scrambling but still nothing comes out of my mouth.

"I think you're just a little naïve, Gavin", Cilla said in a scornful tone. "Sally said she basically wouldn't fancy you if you were pickled". The audience cracks up and I feel like the entire room is focused and laughing directly at me. All 500 eyes burning into me, laughing, ridiculing and mocking the idiot sat on the sofa next to the ultracool Cilla Black, and Sally from Bournemouth.

Finally, my voice appeared, "well I think she still did, Cilla". You think she still did? What? You think she still did? Is that all you could manage, Gav? Is that your best? I mean seriously. Where is the witty retort? Where is the comeback to put Sally down, shut Cilla up and have the audience back on my side?

Scornful remarks aside, Cilla started to warm to me again and said, "well Gavin, its clear that you and Sally weren't a match made in heaven, but what about these thighs I keep hearing about?".

"Sally tell me about these thighs…"

"Oh my god Cilla, he got out the helicopter wearing a pair of cut off denim shorts with these massive tanned thighs", said Sally. I stand up. Time to redeem myself. "You want to see the thighs?" I say to the audience. Standing there strong, hands at the side of my body, palms up. The audience screams, "Yes!!!"

"No, no, no, I can't hear you, I said, do you want to see the thighs?" They scream louder. In one swift motion I grab the waistband of the black trousers I'm wearing and with a fast ripping action forwards, I whip my Velcro trousers off and swing them around my head a few times before throwing them in to the crowd. Redeemed, in one second flat!

These were the Velcro trousers my mum had made for me just a few months ago at the start of my stripping career. Thanks Mum! I digress.

Back to Blind Date. I sit back down on the sofa next to Cilla and Sally. The crowd is cheering still. "Good God, I might take him for myself", said Cilla. The show comes to an end and all the other contestants that were on earlier in the evening come out to sit on the sofa and wave to the crowd. I look down to my boxer shorts and see a little something poking its way through the fly. I smirk to myself. Whether Cilla saw this or not remains to be seen. She never said anything, and I guess we will never know. I've often thought about that moment over the last 25 years and it's never failed to bring a smile to my face.

That was that. That was the time I went on Blind Date and beat Ed Byrne. So, Ed, you have mentioned me many times now, on the radio and TV in various interviews. I only have one thing to say to you: Get over it! You win some, you lose some. You went on to become a famous comedian and I didn't. Them's the breaks; chin up, sweetheart.

The UK Fantasy Boys

Three years later I'm due to graduate. I haven't done any work at university apart from attending a couple of key lectures, but I did drink a lot of beer, eat far too many doner kebabs on the way home from nights out, and make some great friends. I also showed my face to the right lecturers at the right times, but now I have this damn dissertation to write. 10,000 words if I remember correctly.

"There must be a way to get out of it, surely", I think to myself. My prayers are answered a few days later when I get a phone call from a friend called Mark Skipper.

You will recall that I started doing strippograms a few months before I went to uni. Well, my two best mates at the time, Mark Skipper and Tom Dyer, used to come along to my gigs with me. Mostly for fun, but also to meet the girls. It was a win-win for them and me. Anyway, as I left to go to uni, Mark took over my reign as the stripping king of Norfolk and, cutting a very long story short, he'd started working with a stripping troupe called "Obsession" that were based in Manchester. Now he'd come to the decision to form his own troupe consisting of him, myself, Tom Dyer, and Ben Wright; all boys from King's Lynn. We were to be called "The UK Fantasy Boys".

"Gav, how are you mate? Listen, we've got a 12-week tour of Europe coming up and we need 10 guys. I need to know ASAP if you can make it or not. We've got a big promoter in Europe who's seen us perform and he reckons he can sell out some big shows. What do you think?" "Skip, it all sounds great, but I've got four weeks left at uni and a 10,000-word dissertation to start and finish! When exactly do we leave?"

"In 12 days' time". Fuck! I hadn't really enjoyed uni. Didn't feel like I fit in. I'd had happy times there for sure, but it just wasn't me. I hadn't been there for three years to jack my dissertation in at the last minute, but with a promise of 12 weeks gallivanting all over Europe with my best mates, stripping in front of huge crowds and all the trimmings that came with being semi-famous, I must admit, it was very enticing.

"When do you need to know by?" I ask. "By the end of today as I've got more guys than we need all wanting a spot". "I'm in". "That's my man but what about your degree?" "Fuck it".

It sounds amazing and there is no way I'm going to miss out on this. Now all I have to do is convince my parents that this is a good idea and ask my course tutor what my options are. To this day I can't remember what I said to him, but I know it went down like a shit sandwich with Mum and Dad. My course tutor said that I would still graduate, but without honours. "You always have the option to come back and do your dissertation at another time".

I would graduate with not a 1st, a 2nd, not even a Richard the 3rd. Just a bog-standard degree. Oh well. I was off to Europe in less than two weeks for three full months, to perform on stage in front of huge crowds and be paid handsomely for my troubles. I've convinced my tutor and my parents that I'll be back to complete (or rather start) my dissertation sometime in the future, but secretly I know that is never going to happen. I guess they probably do too.

By now you might be wondering, what's that got to do with this book? You might be saying, we know you've been on Blind Date, and you spent the next 16 years working in the stripping industry, travelling all over the UK and Europe, but how is that relevant for me and what's it got to do with this book? How are you even qualified to write this book anyway? Good questions. Allow me to explain.

Everything I've ever done in my life, every experience, every person I've ever met, every single thing, has in some form contributed to the writing of this book. It's the same for every single person on this planet. Think about where you are right now in your life. You made a series of decisions at some point that led to where you are now. It's led you to what you have, and who you are as a person, both good and bad. Wise choices and poor. All these experiences have shaped your life thus far. Everything I've ever done has played a huge part in my life, and I'm grateful for every person, scenario and experience I've had on this journey.

I'd love to tell you more about the stories I've collected from having worked in this amusing and exciting industry for the best part of two decades, but that's another book for another time, and to be honest, I'm not sure I would dare publish it. Now it's time to get serious about the topic at hand.

You will recall that I graduated with some type of sports science degree in 1996. Although my main vocation in life was performing on stage most nights of the week, I realized that I'd probably have to get back into the 'real' world at some point. Throughout these years I was steadily adding more fitness qualifications and skills to my CV, with the view that I would enter that world sooner or later. I got qualified to teach aerobics, step aerobics, body pump, circuit training, boxercise, and spinning. Teaching regular classes each week. I was also doing some personal training with a few clients during the day. I sharpened the sword further by training with industry experts such as Paul Chek and Charles Poliquin and did as much reading as I could around nutrition and fitness.

In February 2008, I travelled to New York with a mate, Ben Wright (UK Fantasy Boys) to attend a fitness/training seminar with the late Mr. Poliquin (RIP) and this event was a huge catalyst for me. In June of the same year, aged 35, I made a bold move. I decided to hang up the G-String and put the baby oil down for good. I retired from stripping. I moved to London to work full-time in the personal training industry. I progressed on to different days, and healthier ways. I will admit it was 13 years later than I'd planned, but that's life sometimes, isn't it? You can make all the best intentions in the world, but sometimes life takes you somewhere entirely unexpected. That's a good thing, in my opinion.

In the last 10 years in central London, I've coached hundreds of clients and delivered over 15,000 hours of one-to-one PT sessions. I've worked with, and coached, clients online from all over the world and invested over £100,000 in my own learning as a coach. I've contributed to various publications like Muscle and Fitness, Men's Health, OK Magazine, Hello Magazine, and The Times newspaper. I've been asked to speak at several events, Lunch and Learns, and various financial institutions in the City. I've taken 40 clients to Ibiza for three fitness retreats.

I've coached ladies and gents, 18 to 70 years old, from every background, religion, race, and social standing. From over 20 different countries, speaking nearly as many languages and all with various desires and goals. I like to think I'm reasonably qualified in this industry, but let's not forget that more importantly perhaps, I was a professional male stripper for 16 years and I've been on "Blind Date" with Cilla Black, Ed Byrne the famous comedian, and Sally from Bournemouth. If you had any doubts as to whether I was qualified to write this book, I'm positive they have now been well and truly quashed. Onwards.

2. THE 80/20 RULE

"Those who ignore the 80/20 rule are doomed to average returns.
Those who use it must bear the burden of exceptional achievement"

- Richard Koch -

In the past if you wanted to know something or find the answer to an obscure question, you'd have to go to the library, find a book, and painstakingly retrieve the answer. Depending on where you lived, this might take a day or even longer, and you'd still have to hunt for the answer. Dr Google has changed our lives in ways we can't even comprehend. We can search and find the answer to literally anything in less than one second. Not only that, but it will give us the answer to an infinite number of questions we may ask around that particular subject. We have information bursting out at the seams. This is both a good and a bad thing. Unfortunately, for all the correct information on the Internet, there is an equal amount of misinformation, which is just as readily available. All you need is a blog and to be able to type, and you're up and running with a presence on the Internet. In the world of health & fitness, it seems everyone has the answer. Every week there is a new fad diet popping up that is the holy grail of weight loss. A brand-new exercise regime that half of Hollywood is following and seeing extraordinary results with.

I just typed "fat loss" into Google and it spouted out 1,060,000,000 websites in 0.40 seconds. I'm not sure I even know how to say that number, but I know it's a lot. Some of it might be relevant and factual, but a lot of it will be just opinions. Even if you find a trusted and reliable source or an expert in this field, there are so many conflicting opinions, as a novice what are you meant to believe? No wonder so many people are confused when it comes to their health & fitness.

I read a study recently that said, "87% of people that go to a gym regularly don't get the results they want". That's an awful statistic when you think about it. It means most people are failing to lose weight, get in shape, and improve their lives. We know that eating a healthy diet, losing weight, and exercising regularly is the best way to stay alive for as long as possible, but most people are failing miserably at this.

If I think back to my younger years when I first fell in love with bodybuilding and weight training back in 1987/88, the only source of information was the odd muscle magazine or the big dude in the gym. I vividly remember performing Arnold Schwarzenegger's "chest routine" three times in one week. "The Oak" famously trained for two hours every day, six days per week. His chest routine consisted of five sets of five exercises with 10 reps per set. This equates to 25 sets & 250 reps in total. Arnold had a big chest and I wanted a big chest, so I copied the routine. I did it for the first time and couldn't move my arms for about three days. "It must be working", I said. I did it again a few days later. Nothing happened. Why wasn't my chest growing? I was a naïve 15-year-old that just wanted to be big and muscular. I didn't realise at the time that Governor Schwarzenegger had been gifted genetically, was using steroids, and his whole life was oriented around training, eating, recovering, and lounging about on Venice beach, California.

I just didn't know that his circumstances were very different to mine. I ploughed on, continuing to fail spectacularly. This is what I see happening all the time in the gym. Many people are trying their best, but performing ineffective exercises and not achieving their goals. Along with the fact that they are eating far too much food, have no real clue how to fuel their body for a workout, never mind how to lose weight and keep it off for good, leaving them stuck and frustrated.

The Pareto principle, also known as the 80/20 rule, states that roughly 80% of the effects come from 20% of the causes. This rule is true in many areas of life, including your health & fitness. Those in the know realise that if you cut out all the nonsense and just do a few key things, you will get tremendous results, with minimal time and effort. Would you believe me if I told you that if you focus on just a couple of key points, you'll get better results than you're currently getting; and probably better than anyone else you know too? Here's the problem. You don't believe it can be that simple. There must be more to it than that, right? It can't be that easy, can it?

It can be, and I'm going to show you how in the coming chapters.

If you're looking for a book with lots of scientific studies, references, and citations, this isn't the book for you. If you're looking for pages and pages of empirical evidence and data, you are in the wrong place. The aim of this book is to cut through all the bullshit on the Internet and dispel a few myths along the way. I'm going to show what works, what doesn't work, and this is all backed by the real-world evidence of what has worked for hundreds of my clients and myself.

I'll show you how to get results even if you have a crazy work schedule, commitments with the family, and just don't know where to start. I'll show you what to focus on and what to discard, and give you all the tried and tested ideas, strategies, and experiential knowledge I've picked up working in the health & fitness industry for over two decades.

Throughout the course of this book, I will refer to several resources that you can download for free and start to use right away. Head over to **www.theghgmethod.com/bonus** to access all the goodies.

3. THE BLUE PILL OR THE RED PILL?

"After this, there is no turning back. You take the blue pill—the story ends, you wake up in your bed and believe whatever you want to believe. You take the red pill—you stay in Wonderland and I show you how deep the rabbit-hole goes. I'm trying to free your mind, Neo"

- Morpheus, "The Matrix" -

The 1999 box office smash hit, "The Matrix" with Keanu Reeves and Laurence Fishburne. What a film. Remember it? Neo (Keanu Reeves) is offered a choice by the rebel leader, Morpheus (Laurence Fishburne). Take the blue pill to have security, happiness, beauty, and the blissful ignorance of illusion. Take the red pill to have knowledge, freedom, uncertainty, and the brutal truths of reality.

The blue pill represented a beautiful prison. Living in ignorance, but without want or fear, in the simulated reality of 'The Matrix'. The red pill offered an uncertain future but the satisfaction of knowing the truth of reality even though it is often harsh and difficult to face. For the purpose of this book, I'm Morpheus, and you are Neo. Just without the long black capes. I'm giving you a choice now. You can take the blue pill and stay exactly where you are right now. Unhappy, overweight and with health problems around the corner, if they aren't here already. Miserable, maybe hating how you look, feeling like you have no energy, and being a poor role model for your children. Comfortable being uncomfortable.

Or, you can take the red pill. The red pill is making a commitment to change. Changing your diet, your health, and ultimately changing your life.

Losing weight and becoming happy, full of energy, pride, and loving life. Becoming a better role model for your family, your children, and yourself. This is by far the harder choice, but the one that ultimately leads to fulfilment and greatness.

What's it going to be? The blue pill or the red pill? Choose wisely my friend. Your life literally depends on it. If you chose the blue pill, you should put this book down right now. It won't help you. No hard feelings, but your time will be best spent elsewhere. If you chose the red pill, I salute you. You've just made one of the toughest decisions there is to make. The great thing is, you won't regret it for a second, and you won't ever look back. Metaphors aside, you can decide in a heartbeat, "enough is enough. I need to make changes and they start right here, now, today".

Still reading? Great. That means you took the right path. Welcome. Your life officially gets better from here on in.

Firstly, I want to tell you about an old client of mine. We'll call him Jim, because that was his name. He was receiving my daily emails for the best part of two years. He told me when he started working with me that he sat on the fence for two years saying, "I must do something about this". He knew he was 40lbs overweight and that his life wasn't where he wanted it to be. Ultimately, he was the one who had to email me, pull the trigger, take action, and join my programme. Something he read one morning in one of my emails was the straw that broke the camel's back. Whatever it was spurred him on to finally respond to the email. He joined my coaching programme and I helped him lose 40lbs and never find them again.

Jim was a classic example of someone who was in a lot of pain and knew he needed to make some big changes in his life. Jim chose the red pill, but it took him two years to make a decision. Tony Robbins says, "We all get what we tolerate". Many people are comfortable enough being uncomfortable that they don't do anything about it, which is an awful scenario to be in.

I know you might be sitting there thinking, "I don't even know where to start, I don't know how to do this, and I just haven't got time". Guess what? Everyone's busy and most people don't know what to do. Read on. You've got to this point. You've picked up my book. You've made a decision. You actually want to pull the trigger. Read to the end of this book and I promise I won't let you down. Let's make some real differences to your health and ultimately your life. You took the red pill remember?

4. THE GHG METHOD

"There's a method to my madness; and a madness to my method"

- Salvador Dali -

Now you might be wondering what the hell "GHG" stands for. It's a good question. The 2 G's? That's Gavin Gillibrand. I'm sure you guessed that. The H stands for Howard but keep that to yourself, please. Thanks.

There are a myriad of diets, training plans and fitness regimes that are all available for FREE on the Internet to download right now, so why listen to me? What makes my ideas and philosophies stand out? Over the last 20 years in this business, I've tried everything you can think of. Programmes, training schedules, and diets. Every "supplement", legal and illegal, I've given it a whirl, all in the attempt to grow big muscles, get a six-pack and stay strong, fit, and healthy.

A lot of what I've tried didn't work. Some of it did and what I've come to realise over these years is that body and health transformations are like baking a cake. You need a recipe and you need to follow it. Miss one key ingredient and the cake is a mess. Stray from the recipe and add additional ingredients, you end up with a completely different cake. You can have a great training programme but if your diet is poor, you get poor results. Your diet looks good and your training schedule is great, but you have no consistency, guess what? Your results will be poor. Maybe you are training hard, eating healthy but your sleep is terrible. This will hamper your progress.

A combination of exercise, nutrition, success habits, and the correct mindset is vital to achieve great results. Even more importantly, maintain them and never go back to where you started. Throughout this book, you will see a small snapshot of some of the clients I've had the pleasure of working with. Clients like Kenny who lost 27lbs working with me over a period of 12 weeks. Lane lost 28lbs. Kevin lost 29.5lbs. Jason lost 30.5lbs. All in 12 weeks. Jim lost 40lbs in 5 months. The list goes on. I've helped hundreds of clients lose weight and transform their health and life using my methodologies. Are they perfect? No. Nothing is. But they are practical, sustainable, and easy to implement. Above all, my clients have fun on the way, which is what you want, isn't it?

We all know there's more than one way to skin a cat. Over 20 years in this game and years of being a human guinea pig have allowed me to cut the wheat from the chaff so to speak and bring this book to you. I hope you enjoy reading it.

Welcome to The GHG Method.

5. JUST WHERE THE HELL ARE YOU?

"Now is the only reality. All else is either memory or imagination"

- Osho -

Look at where you are right now with your health, body, and fitness. Don't sugar coat it, but don't condemn yourself either. If you don't know where you are right now, how are you going get to where you want to go? Stand naked in front of a full-length mirror. It's a sobering thought for many, but it might be just what you need. That's the harsh reality staring back at you. The sooner you accept it, the sooner you can make some changes.

Many people will avoid doing this and bury their head in the sand like an ostrich, which is believed (incorrectly I might add) to hide its head in a hole in the ground when it sees danger. If ostriches did bury their heads in the sand (they don't), I'd say, don't be an ostrich. The awareness of where you are right now is very important. Acknowledge, "I'm in this situation right now and this is where I need to change". Accept where you are in terms of your health, your fitness, how your body looks, and how you feel. It can be painful but also very liberating.

Former Navy SEAL turned best selling author Jocko Willink talks about this in his book, *"Extreme Ownership"*. Extreme ownership is taking control and accepting exactly where you are right now. In other words saying, "There's no one else to blame but myself for exactly the position I'm in right now. I'm going to take full responsibility for where I am with my health, where I am with my fitness, where I am with my life, then I'm going to make the necessary changes to move my life to where I want it to be". All the decisions you've ever made have led you to where you are in this moment. You are 100% responsible for your health, and your life. Accepting and being OK with that can be a tough but important moment for many.

Where are you? Do you have 20, 30, 40lbs to lose? More maybe? Do you get out of breath going up the stairs or walking up a hill? Is the waistband on your trousers tight and restrictive? Do you have a favourite suit jacket that you can't wear anymore? Are you in pain from sitting at your desk all day? Are you tired, lethargic, and irritable? Do you go to sleep wired and wake up exhausted? What exactly are your physical symptoms?

Let's look at this from the inside, as well as the outside.

Do you hate how you look and feel when you look in the mirror? Do you feel disgusted with your own body? Like you have so much more potential inside? Do you feel like you're letting your family down and even more importantly perhaps, letting yourself down? Are you happy in life or are you depressed? Do you wake up each day and jump out of bed with energy, drive, and motivation; or do you hit snooze several times and wish you could stay in bed a little longer? Do you relish the day ahead or do you wish it would just end so you could retreat into the warmth and safety of that cosy pit of yours?

To be honest, you may not know exactly how you feel because no one has ever asked you before. You likely have not asked yourself these questions. You just have an underlying, overwhelming feeling of negativity and discontent. Maybe.

Maybe you know exactly how you feel and exactly what you want and need to change. If so, that's good. Maybe you are disgusted with how you look AND feel. Maybe you've had a health scare and a reality check from the doctor? Or maybe you're just sick to the back teeth of feeling like shit? Hold that feeling. You're going to need those feelings and emotions if you ever hope to make some serious life-long changes.

Writing about how you feel on paper can be helpful for some. Experiments have shown that people who write about emotionally charged episodes experience a marked increase in their physical and mental wellbeing. Write below the three words that come to the forefront of your mind when you think about where you are with your current level of health & fitness. Don't worry about feeling stupid. I've found that the people that interact the most in exercises like this tend to gain the most benefit.

E.G. You might be feeling frustrated, disappointed, and fed up. You may be feeling depressed, demotivated, and angry. Write how you feel in three words below. Don't rush. Have a good think. Take your time.

1:

_____

2:

_____

3:

_____

I don't know if writing down how you feel has made you feel better, but it probably hasn't made you feel worse. You might be even more determined to do something now you've recognised exactly how you feel. Be honest with yourself. We can make a start from there.

Working with clients

I can ask a client to tell me how they feel, but to really know where they're at I need a few basic details that will give me a bigger picture. I always ask for a seven-day food and drink diary. Everything they eat and drink, good and bad, for a week. This gives me a great idea of not only what they eat, but also how they eat: timings, quantities, and habits. Plus, it will show the difference between weekdays and the weekend, which for most people is when things go horribly wrong. A detailed food and drink diary will give me a great snapshot of their life. It will tell me whether food and nutrition is important to that person, a case of convenience, or maybe even just an afterthought. Success in the coaching game is won and lost on the ability of the client to adhere to basic nutritional principles. It doesn't mean eating like a rabbit for weeks on end, nor does it mean severe restriction like many people believe. It simply relies on a few basic rules.

I ask the client to weigh him/herself. Weight is an important benchmark that will be monitored throughout the time I work with a client. If someone has a lot of weight to lose, we obviously want that scale to be shifting south, but it's not the be all and end all. No one knows what you weigh. You don't walk around with a sign on the front of your head saying, "I weigh 15 stone". The truth is, we don't know what that end number will be. The aim is to burn body fat and build, or at least preserve, lean muscle tissue. Body composition is our goal. That means we want a favourable ratio of LBM (lean body mass) to adipose tissue (body fat).

I like to have the client take pictures or have pictures taken of them in underwear or swimwear. One picture from the front, one from the side, and one from the rear. This is uncomfortable for most. Understandably of course, which is one of the reasons I ask them to do it. Firstly, a visual record of the starting point, week-to-week progress, and the end result is very powerful for the client and helps me. Secondly, asking the client to step out their comfort zone, by taking a picture or three of themselves semi-naked and sending them to their coach, is very empowering.

A picture is worth a thousand words, the old idiom states, and in this case it's never been truer. Very often a client will be visibly shocked when we compare the picture from week 1 next to the picture in week 12. Shocked in a positive way. When you see yourself day in and day out, it's hard to notice the difference. You know things are working, but when you drop 20-30lbs over a three-month period, the visual difference is phenomenal when you look back at it.

Next up are measurements. With a tape measure and the help of someone, I like to have the following measurements:

- Chest
- Upper waist
- Lower waist
- Hips (female)
- Non-dominant upper arm
- Non-dominant upper leg (quads)

Measurements, like pictures, are very tangible and simply don't lie. When a client sees that they're losing inches on paper, it's very encouraging. This can be invaluable if the scales haven't moved much and the client is perhaps feeling disappointed. With the loss of inches, the client's outlook is much more positive than only using the weight on the scale as an indicator of success.

When a client sees these starting measurements and pictures - the cold hard facts of where they are right now with their health & fitness - it can go one of two ways. It's a real leveler for many and an eye-opener. It can send the client away inspired, motivated, and ready to make some big changes in their life. "This is where I am. Shit. No one else to blame, this is all me. I'm here, this is real and it's up to me to change". Or it can have the opposite effect entirely. I've seen clients throw the towel in before we even begin. The stark reality of their current situation has been too much for them to handle, but it's a necessary process that you must go through if you're to create the results you desire. It's a punch in the face, but not one from which you can't recover.

Lane was a client of mine a while back. He was a big lad with a lot of weight to lose. He weighed 22 stone and even though he was 6'3 tall, I figured he had at least five stone to lose before he was anything close to being healthy. I asked him to weigh himself and send me some pictures. I didn't need to know any measurements. It just wasn't necessary and under these circumstances, I felt it would only cause more anguish to an already delicate situation. Lane had been thinking of working with me for over a year before he plucked up the courage to pick up the phone. I wasn't going to do anything to make him feel more uncomfortable than he already was. I asked him if he was OK with the pictures and he assured me he was.

As we worked together, we looked at three areas to gauge his improvement. His weight, his pictures, and his performance in the gym. The scales were moving in the right direction and his performance in the gym was going up (an increase in the weights being lifted), so I knew that progress was being made. From that alone, I knew it was unlikely he was losing any muscle mass and he was definitely burning body fat. This, coupled with regular photos, showed us both that he was losing a tonne of body fat and his shape was changing rapidly. Lane went on to lose over two stone (29lbs) with me in just 12 weeks and increased his bench press, deadlift, and squat significantly, which he was most surprised by.

Go to **www.theghgmethod.com/bonus** to download the free checklist on how to take your measurements correctly.

Lane's testimonial:

"I have always struggled with my weight (and suffered with an overactive knife and fork). I had always done a lot of weightlifting but had never taken the nutrition seriously – I had thought that to lose weight I'd have to basically become vegan and live on lentils and sunflower seeds. I was also afraid I wouldn't be as strong if I lost weight, but 12 weeks later and over two stone lighter, I couldn't be happier. I eat a lot of high protein/low carb foods, which means I'm always full up and I'm not losing muscle. I can now deadlift and bench press more than ever. I couldn't have done this without Gav's

knowledge, experience, and his 12-week coaching plan – he gave me a plan to follow, I did just that and it worked. If anyone were considering getting a coach, I'd recommend working with Gav 100%.

6. MOTIVATION

"When you feel like quitting, think about "why" you started"

- Unknown -

Very often, I speak to prospective clients that say, "I know what to do, I just need help with motivation". This could be true to a certain extent and there is no doubt that you need motivation to begin. To decide, "Enough is enough" and start exercising or eating in a way that will produce results to improve your health.

That's great, but what are you going to do when you're not motivated? Motivation tends to be high for exercise when the other areas of your life are going well. When your work and family life are running smoothly, motivation is much easier. When the cogs of life are turning nicely, it's easy to get out of bed at 5am and go to the gym before work. When life is challenging, it's not so easy. If your sleep is devastated because your son or daughter was sick in the night, your motivation will likely be very low in the morning. You get a roasting from your boss and it wasn't your fault. This could motivate you more to get to the gym or it could push you in the direction of the pub or sofa. There are so many ups and downs in the course of life that if you rely on the ups to motivate you, then you will surely fail when you go through the downs.

I've found that even the most highly motivated individuals lack motivation at some point in their life. In fact, if you were to ask many professional athletes if they feel motivated to train all the time, they would say they don't. So, what makes some people seem "motivated" and others not? It's not motivation. Motivation is a finite resource. It runs out. For some, it's much sooner than others. I believe there are a few key factors to achieving success in any endeavour. Firstly, clarity on what you want to achieve. Secondly, a bloody good reason why you want to achieve that goal and what it will mean to you if/when you achieve it. Finally, you need a plan; preferably one that works.

Clarity

Most people don't even know what they want to achieve. "I want to lose weight" won't really do. How much weight do you want to lose? How many pounds do you want to lose? You need some real clarity here. Give me an exact number please. If you don't specify precisely what you want, how the hell do you think you will achieve it, and how will you know if you've been successful? If you go on a diet and lose 2lbs is that a success? You've lost weight, but I would guess for most people, that wouldn't be classed as a successful result.

Your "Why"

Let's say your goal is to lose two stone or nearly 30lbs. Why do you want to lose that weight? It's not the weight that you are interested in; it's what you obtain from having lost that weight. How do you want to look and feel? Why do you want to look and feel like that? What does that mean to you? How will your life improve? How will others engage and react to you? Why is all this important to you? Simon Sinek talks about it in his book "*It starts with WHY*".

Your 'Why' is the reason you get out of bed everyday and work towards that goal. Your 'Why' is the reason you sacrifice things in your life like television or going out drinking with friends. It's the underlying basis of an overarching desire that pulls you towards the success you want to obtain. You can keep pushing and use motivation but when motivation wanes, an even greater force is pulling you forward. The people that see real success on a huge level have a strong sense of why. When things get tough - and they will get tough - you will want to quit. That's normal so don't stress over it. In fact, if you don't want to quit, you're not working hard enough. If it's all plain sailing you're not pushing the boundaries of what could be. You're not driving hard enough. Things need to be uncomfortable. Scrap that. Things need to be bloody tough. You want to quit. You're not sure that you're good enough, not sure you can make it. You may run out of motivation, energy, and all-round determination to succeed; but with a huge

'Why' it becomes easy. Actually, it's never easy. It becomes easier. As though something is pulling you towards your goal like a magnet. Mix this with a little motivation to get you going in the beginning and you're on your way. Your 'Why' must be SO strong that nothing will deter you from working towards that goal. Whatever the obstacle or whatever the set back, you keep working towards what you want to achieve. Nothing can get in your way. You almost feel invincible. Your goal is non-negotiable. It's not something that you "might" work towards; there is something powerful driving you towards it. It's inevitable that you will achieve it. You get up in the morning knowing that shit is gonna get done.

That's the feeling you want to have when you have a goal. That's the energy and drive you need if you want to succeed. I'm not saying you can't achieve things without a huge 'Why'. You can, but you can achieve far greater success, far quicker, and with much more impact, if you have that invisible force pulling you, dragging you towards where you want to be.

What is Your 'Why?'

My 'Why' for everything in my life is based around my children. I have two. One daughter aged 14 (going on 19), called Mia, and a baby boy who just turned 15 months, Gabriel. These two are the reason I get up at 5am every day and work hard at whatever I'm doing. Kids, as I'm sure you all know, learn from what we do rather than what we say to them. They're always watching. I work hard to be the best father to them and the best role model that I can be, so they grow up proud of their old man. My hope is that they take the best that I have and use that to propel them to even greater heights in their own life. It's both exciting and scary to know that the things I do in my life are literally shaping theirs.

How to Find Your "Why"

A lot of people say, "I don't know my reason why". Here is a very simple but effective exercise you can do right now. Grab a pen and paper.

Start by clearly stating your objective or goal. Let's say you want to lose 30lbs.

Ask "why?". Your answer might be: "So I can fit into some of my old clothes that are several sizes smaller". Make sure you write that down.

Ask "why?" again: "So I can be more attractive and confident".

Why? What would being more attractive and confident give you?

Keep asking why as many times as you need to get to the real reason you want to lose weight. It may surprise you. Very often the real reason is different to the reason you openly say. Losing weight is not about the number on the scales. It's what that number gives you. Better health, energy, confidence, better relationships, and so on.

A Plan That Works

You're motivated and have a burning desire. You have a whopping great 'WHY'. Is success guaranteed? Nope. What? Why not? You can have all this but even more important than that is having the skills and a well thought out plan to execute. Highly motivated, with a massive 'WHY', but no skills and no plan; you won't achieve anything.

"Motivation is fine but without a plan and with no skills, all you end up with is a motivated idiot", says Tony Robbins.

Now I'm not calling you an idiot and I'm sure Tony isn't either, but you get the point, I hope. You can be highly motivated with a great work ethic and achieve very little if you spend your time doing the wrong things. I often see people in the gym working very hard but performing ineffective exercises that just don't produce results. This will ultimately lead to frustration and the classic, "it doesn't work for me" or, "I can't lose weight, whatever I try". A professional athlete won't get results either, if they perform the wrong exercises, however strong their why and the clarity of their goals.

7. WHERE DO YOU WANT TO BE?

"A goal is a dream with a deadline"

- Napoleon Hill -

We've established where you currently are. It's the first step on this journey to success. Now we need to look at where you want to go. What are your goals? It's extremely important to have a goal and write that down. It's a cliché, but you can't hit a goal that you can't see.

Why Set Goals?

Studies show that you're 24 times more likely to achieve a goal if you write it down. Yet most people don't set goals. In fact, a recent study suggested that 97% of people have never written their goals down. Many people set New Year's resolutions and we all know what happens there, don't we? In January the gyms across the country are packed with people full of good intentions. By the end of February, the gyms are back to normal. Business as usual. The good intentions have died a quick and painful death. These resolutions mean nothing, which is why most people fail. They're just dreams and wishes. The average person doesn't set any goals and I'm assuming you would rather not be average? That said, let's get into it.

Your Goal Must Be Specific

You must state what you want. Don't be afraid of saying exactly what you want to achieve. Many people are quite scared to say what they want for fear of being perceived as selfish. In this case, you're entitled to think for yourself. Scrap that. In this situation, it's a must.

"I want to lose weight" will not do. The brain likes details and will respond best when given a direct command. "I want to lose 30lbs" is far more powerful. A vague thought or comment about losing weight is just a dream or a wish. Dreams don't come true. Strong powerful goals that are executed do.

Accountability

Share your goal with someone you respect, who will hold you to it. This is very powerful. This person will hold your feet to the fire. The very act of sharing your goal makes you work harder to achieve it, purely to not be seen as a failure in front of this person. However, a word of warning; be careful whom you share your goals and dreams with. Be very sure that this person will encourage you and actually want you to achieve your goals. Many people, and often the people closest to us, act like they want us to achieve great things but in reality, it can make them feel very uncomfortable.

That person has choices. They go with you as you become successful on your health or weight loss journey, which might mean they lose weight with you, or they support and encourage you every step of the way, regardless of where they are with their own health, fitness, and weight. Alternatively, they stay where they are as you move forward. The gap between you gets wider. It's not a physical gap, it's a mental one, but it's real, nonetheless. This gap can become extremely difficult for the person who stays the same and whether they realise it or not, they might start trying to pull you back. This happens subconsciously and often, they're not even aware they're doing it.

"You've lost enough weight now, don't get too skinny".

They think they've got your best interests at heart. Maybe they have, and they're simply misguided. Sometimes it can be a lot more blatant.

"You won't lose 30lbs, you've always been fat" or, "Don't be silly. You will never lose that weight".

Sometimes these comments from the people we love the most can cripple our confidence and stop us before we even begin. The doubts can creep in:

"Well, maybe you're right…I can't do that…"

Get Rid of Your Crabs

Many people have what is known as a "crab mentality". If you look at a bucket of crabs you will see one or two ambitious crabs on the top, desperately trying with all their might to get out over the edge of the bucket. The crabs below will do everything they can to stop that one crab leaving. The "If I'm not getting out, neither are you" type of mentality. It's a common attitude for many. Don't buy into THEIR insecurities and jealousy. You CAN achieve your goal, with or without that person in your corner. Find the right person who will support you every step of the way and simply don't talk about it with anyone who you think will not be supportive.

Write, Read and Visualise That Goal Daily

This is the toughest one for most. Hands up if you've ever written your weight loss goal down on paper? Obviously, I can't see you, but I'd bet that most of you didn't raise your hand. The R.A.S or "reticular activating system" is a mechanism in the brain that dictates your level of awareness toward a certain subject. Have you ever bought a new car? It arrives and you're so proud of it. Taking it for a spin and to your utter dismay every second car you see is the same as yours? How annoying is this? You're now blatantly aware of this make and model of car and suddenly see it everywhere. That's your R.A.S. "looking" out for it.

Every day, we are bombarded with thousands of adverts, messages, thoughts, emails, and updates. We'd go mad trying to process all this information. Your brain is incredibly clever and filters out the "junk" that isn't important. Those cars were always visible; you just didn't see them, as they weren't "front of mind".

By writing, reading and saying aloud your goal it tells your brain that this is important. Resources, people, scenarios, and things appear to show up and help in reaching your destination. It's not magic. They were always there but now you're open to receiving "the magic" that is all around. It's extremely powerful. It's almost like a reverse conspiracy. Stuff just seems to go right all the time. Read your goal out loud first thing in the morning and last thing at night, just before you sleep. Your subconscious mind gets to work on it and often you will wake up with new ideas and inspiration to help you move forward and achieve your goal.

I've got a great tip for you when it comes to writing your goal down. Write it on a piece of paper and stick it to the fridge. Why on the fridge? Because it will remind you when you go to get some food. "This is my goal". It's a little mental cue that can steer you in the right direction when you're about to make a bad decision on your diet. It could be the difference between reaching for a bottle of water instead of the bottle of Budweiser and going for the Greek yoghurt when you really fancy a salted caramel ice cream bar from Häagen-Dazs. By the way, I'm talking to myself here as much as you.

A Date and a Deadline

Linked closely to point number one. "I want to lose 30lbs by June 1st". In fact, what's even better is stating, "I weigh 30lbs less on June 1st" or, "I weigh 170lbs on June 1st". Specificity and a deadline are a must.

When you set a date, good things happen. That's not to say you don't have to work hard, of course you do. Just by setting the date you will not miraculously achieve your goal, but when you do set the date and deadline, you have a far greater chance of achieving your goal because whether you realise it or not, your subconscious mind gets to work helping you achieve it. You go to bed with your goal in mind, you wake up with your goal in your thoughts, and throughout the day, this deadline will steer you and keep you on the correct path towards it.

Expect it to Happen

You must believe you can achieve your goal. Many people set goals that are too unrealistic to achieve in the given time frame. You don't need to know how just yet, but you must believe that you can achieve it. You must believe it's possible. The how is irrelevant for now.

You can achieve pretty much any goal you want if you work hard and long enough on it but so many people that set goals, set ones that are beyond their capabilities in the time frame they allow. Never change the goal but change the deadline. Some guy says, "I want to lose five stone in eight weeks". It's an ambitious goal for sure and it's not going to be possible, unless we take his leg off at the hip. I'm not an advocate of amputation for weight loss.

Make the goals lofty but not so far beyond normal comprehension that you know in your heart you will never, ever achieve it. I'm 5'8 tall on a good day. 5'10 if I wear my Cuban heels. If my goal were to dunk a basketball, I'd have my work cut out. With all things considered, the odds are against me. Why? Because I'm 5'8 and 6'4 is small in basketball. Having said that, I saw Nate Robinson playing for the New York Jets at Madison Square Garden a few years ago, dunking all over his opponents and he is 5'8.

Wesley Snipes said, "White men can't jump". That's cool because this one has no desire to, but if it was really important to me, is it possible that I could dunk a basketball? Yes, of course it's *possible*, but I'd probably have to spend my entire life working towards that goal and I would require a burning desire to make it happen. As I said before, you never change the goal. You only change the deadline. These points are vital to think about when writing your goals, but the most important factor in my opinion, is having a big, fat compelling reason 'why'.

A few years ago, in my days of personal training, I had a client called Matt. Matt had been training with me for about six months, but he wasn't getting the results he wanted. He'd be the first to admit that this was because he wasn't following his diet as well as he might have. The weekends were his downfall. We had never set goals when we first started training together, but with his wedding just six months away, it was time to get serious. "I just want to be ripped for Ibiza and the wedding", he said.

We set three-month and six-months goals. He wrote these down, committing pen to paper. He did all the things I said above about putting his goal on the fridge. He told his partner, for accountability, who was incredibly supportive. In the next six months he lost 21 pounds of body fat and became ripped with a six-pack. He arrived in Ibiza in the shape of his life, happier than ever, and ready to marry the man of his dreams. To be honest, Matt's results were some of the best I've ever had the pleasure of being a part of. Much of the success came down to proper goal setting.

Matt's testimonial:

"Wow. I've never expected to have such dramatic before and after photos. I'm extremely pleased with the results. Gav helps you tweak your diet to ratchet up the results. He knows when to push and when to back off and always does it with his trademark sense of humour. If you're undecided about whether to be coached by Gav, just go for it. Follow his advice and watch the results start to happen from the

*outset. **We decided to get serious, set some real goals and I've been blown away with the results. I can now go to Ibiza knowing I've never looked or felt this great.***"

Many people don't write goals down because they think, "I've got the goal in my head and that's enough". The physical act of writing your goals down, putting pen to paper, is extremely powerful.

Everything is a choice. You can choose to take the advice of someone who has done this hundreds of times or you can decide not to do it. It can be tedious committing that goal to paper, but if it meant losing 40 pounds or achieving the results that you want to; all those things you mentioned about feeling great, feeling energized, having the kids respect you, being a great role model for your children; wouldn't it be worth it?

Go to **www.theghgmethod.com/bonus** for an abbreviated goal setting cheat sheet and checklist that you can print out and pin to your fridge.

8. ROADBLOCKS & RESISTANCE

"Smooth seas do not make skillful sailors"

- African proverb -

It's important to know the potential roadblocks that may appear because if you recognise them early and expect them, you're far better equipped to deal with them. It's all very well knowing where you are and having a goal, but you may be thinking that you're a special case...

"My situation is very, very different to everyone else, you just don't understand. I'm extremely busy at work. I've got kids. My boss doesn't let me go to the gym. I travel all the time. I don't even get a lunch break. Weekends are family time".

Fill in your own personal favourite. I get it. You're busy. You can't allow yourself to use that as an excuse. Actually, you can, but you shouldn't. Don't do it. Everyone is busy. We all get the same 24 hours in the day. What you need to realise is that you're always going have these roadblocks. There's always going to be things that get in the way.

The physical roadblocks from circumstances and the mental resistance, which are usually bullshit stories imagined in your head. Being aware of these potential roadblocks that could stop you, you can take the necessary measures to avoid them in the first place by planning and preparing things, or at least be able to deal with them when they arise.

Very often I have clients come to me and say, "I can work with you over the next 12 weeks because I've literally got nothing in the diary". I tell them,

"Are you kidding me? You must be the most boring person in the world because if you haven't got stuff in the diary for the next 12 weeks, your life must be pretty dull. Come back to me when you've got a life".

Joking aside, I don't necessarily say it that way. However, you're always going have stuff in the diary. Children are going to get sick. Your train is going be late. Christmas happens every year. The boss is going ask you to spend more time at work. You might be the boss, in which case you might be working even more. There's always going to be stuff that gets in the way of having a smoothly running, perfect life, because a perfect life doesn't exist. It doesn't exist for me and doesn't exist for you. Please realise that shit will always happen and know that every other person reading this book who wants to achieve similar results, is going to have the same shit happen to them too. We're all human beings trying to get results. By recognising the fact that "things" can and will go wrong, you can plan and prepare for them.

Let's say you set the alarm early. You've got to get to work at your normal time but you've allowed a 90-minute time window to get to the gym, get back, shower, have breakfast, and be back out the door to work. That's the perfect scenario if you choose to go to the gym or do some exercise before work. However, the new baby in the house was up three times in the night - because that's what babies do - and your sleep has been completely decimated for the night. The alarm goes off at 5.30am and you realise you probably had four hours of sleep, if you're lucky.

Now you have two choices. You can go to the gym, extremely tired and think, "screw it, I'm going to do it anyway" or you could allow that situation to completely mess up your plans. Very often you're going to choose the latter. That's not because you're weak, it's because it's very tiring to go to the gym and do a full day's work when you've only had three-or four-hours kip. That doesn't make you a bad person. That makes you human. The chances of that happening, if you've got young children are very high.

At the time of writing this book, I had a meeting with someone in the diary for 9am one morning. I had planned to hit the gym early and be ready for my meeting by 9. My baby son, Gabriel was up three times in the night and although I didn't get out of bed, Alex, my fiancée did, I was awake for at least 20 to 30 minutes each time, so my sleep was wrecked for the night. I was late for my first meeting in the morning as I overslept and didn't make the gym. I was annoyed at this but realised that things will always happen. I did manage to get to the gym later in the day, despite being knackered. I choose that path instead of the path of least resistance. I didn't want to. It would have been far easier to sack off the gym and get home for a nice home-cooked meal, but my goal was to go to the gym, so I made it happen. I'm not saying that this has always happened and always will happen. But in this instance it did. My resolve was strong, and I took THAT path instead of the easy path that led to the sofa and Netflix. "The path with the most resistance always leads to greatness", said Ryan Holiday in his book *"The Obstacle is the Way"*.

You've got a PT session booked tonight and you're just about to finish for the day. You're tidying up the papers on your desk, shutting your computer down, just about to go out the door for a gym session and the boss calls you in and says, "I need you to get that report done for tomorrow. We've got a client arriving at 9am". Now you're stuck at the office for the next two hours to finish the report. You can mutter under your breath all the expletives you want, and you probably do, but it's not going to change the situation. PT session gone. Lost money and time. Bloody frustrating. Do you let that situation completely derail you or do you have a contingency plan in place? "Okay, I didn't manage to go to the gym today. Maybe I can get an extra session in at the weekend?"

If you've still managed to train twice this week and you miss the third time, do you think to yourself, "in the grand scheme of things, is this gonna affect my results?" or do you think what many people think, "I've missed my gym session, so screw it. I'll eat a load of crap food tonight and have a drink to feel better about it"?

Maybe you were really prepared and cooked your food to take into work. You cooked dinner the night before and made extra food so there was a portion left over for your wife and another for you to take into work the next day. It's sitting in a Tupperware container in the fridge. You race out the door in the morning, as you're late for the train. Damn! You've left your food in the fridge. Now you've got three choices. You could rush back, but chances are you won't do that. You could think, "Screw it. There goes my healthy lunch" and just eat some of the crap that's local to you, or you could go to Marks & Spencer's and make a healthy food choice, while committing to remember your lunch tomorrow. No big deal.

My point is this: there are going to be scenarios, situations, and things that will happen which seemingly stop you from achieving your results. It's what you do about these situations that counts. The decisions you make in these moments; are you going to be proactive or reactive? Proactive means you will accept the situation, as it is, perhaps even have a plan B, and act accordingly. Link it with your goal and your 'why'. Reactive is living in the moment and making a poor decision, almost to spite yourself. This will only take you further away from your goal. It is perhaps even a method of self-sabotage to maintain our former "identity". Humans are strange and complex beings.

Some of you will be thinking, "I'm different. You don't understand my situation. I'm busier than most", etc. This takes me back to the quote I mentioned from Jocko Willink in *"Extreme Ownership"*. Take ownership of exactly where you are with your life right now. You might think you're busier than others and you've got more problems than others but let me say that everyone has the same stuff going on in their lives, in different ways. We've all got the same 24 hours in the day.

The best way to overcome these situations is to not beat yourself up. Accept that these situations are normal, and they may happen. Have a contingency plan in place. It's a realisation that shit happens, and it's how you deal with the shit that is important. Do you let it completely throw you off path from the goals you're trying to achieve, or do you accept it in your stride, move past it, and carry on with your day? Accepting where you are, that you face the same problems as everyone else and moving past those tough situations is the way you succeed with anything in life.

Grab a pen and piece of A4 paper. Time to do a little work. Don't skip this bit, it's important.

Welcome to the SWOT analysis. SWOT is an acronym for strengths, weaknesses, opportunities, and threats. On your sheet of paper, draw a line down the middle from top to bottom. Now draw a line from left to right half way down the page. You should now have four compartments. Four quarters of the page. In the top left space write the word "Strengths". Top right hand, write the word "Weaknesses". Bottom left, write the word "Opportunities" and in the bottom right, write the word "Threats".

In each box, write down three of each. For example, in the "strengths" box you could write:

1. Good timekeeper. 2. Highly motivated. 3. Gym in my office building (no excuse)

Go through each area and write down five in each box. In fact, start with five but list as many as you can in each section. The aim of this exercise is to establish exactly where you are and look at what may go wrong. You can identify some of the potential roadblocks. Recognise them early and avoid them. The upside to this is you will identify all the things that are in your favour. Things you may have not realised. It's a very valuable exercise; so take 10 minutes to fill this in.

Here's a visual of what I mean:

Strengths	Weaknesses
1. 2. 3. 4. 5.	1. 2. 3. 4. 5.
Opportunities 1. 2. 3. 4. 5.	**Threats** 1. 2. 3. 4. 5.

A Contingency Plan

Let's say your programme says to go to the gym on a Monday and for some reason, Monday turned out to be a horrendous day. No chance of getting to the gym as you arrive home after 8pm. Do you sack it off entirely, eat crappy food, and grab a beer from the fridge or do you do what you can with the time available? Perhaps a 15-20-minute body-weight workout that can be performed in your bedroom would keep you progressing towards your goals, both mentally and physically? Is it your intended workout? No. Is it as good as what you had planned? Possibly not, but you've adapted and overcome an annoying situation and made the most of it – that's what winners do. They overcome, adapt and move forwards, just like my client Kevin did.

Kevin was extremely busy with work and family commitments. He was doing very well with his nutrition but couldn't seem to find time to get the scheduled workouts in the diary. He was beating himself up because of this. I asked what he could commit to each week? He said "3 x 30 minutes". So that's what he did. He wasn't doing the prescribed workouts with the frequency that would have been optimal, but we had to reach a point that was manageable and sustainable for him. We did that, as you will see from his testimonial below.

Kevins Testimonial:

"After a health checkup, I knew I had to change. I am 47 and weighed 18 stone. After a couple of chats with Gav, I came to the realisation that it was much more than weight loss that I needed. I needed a change in mindset and how my body works. Gav gave me a plan and explained why I had to follow the plan. Gav imparted knowledge regarding nutrition and exercise through his coaching calls, in a way that it made sense and encouraged me to adopt a new way of thinking. On his 12-week coaching programme I lost 13.5kg of body fat. I feel fitter and healthier than I have done for years.

Yes, I know, you're thinking this can't be true. If you'd told me I would lose that much body fat in three months I would never have believed you, but it is just through understanding what your body requires and sound nutritional advice that works, but something that is easy to follow and manageable. If you are sitting on the fence, undecided about whether to get a coach or not, my advice would be to get off the fence and on the phone. Call Gav, he will help you".

Wise words from Kevin, but then I would say that, wouldn't I?

9. FACE YOUR FEARS

"Love is what we are born with. Fear is what we learn"

- Buddha -

As babies we come into this world with only two fears. These are the fear of falling and the fear of loud noises. The rest are learned behaviours that we adopt and take from our environment, our parents, or a negative situation that occurred at some point in our lives. In many cases, they're totally irrational. Things like public speaking, spiders, fear of flying, and heights are the common fears that many people have. I think you must have a healthy respect for certain things but when it sets a person into a panic, it has passed over into being irrational. If you want to succeed in most areas of life the process will be scary. You don't want to take that first step. Fear of failure, fear of something that might go wrong, and fear of success even. Sometimes you just have to jump in with both feet.

I like to use the acronym F.E.A.R. False. Evidence. Appearing. Real. Or in some cases, it appears to be Fuck Everything And Run. Comfort zones eh? You know that nice, cosy place we all love to be, in every aspect of our lives. The comfort zone is the complete opposite of stepping into the things we fear. Unfortunately, it's what holds us all back in achieving what we truly desire. We've all got at least one thing we're fearful of. Some have many more and it can stop you from taking action when you really want to. What are you fearful of? What are you scared of? What are your insecurities? I will show you mine, if you show me yours. (Get your mind out of the gutter, please).

I'm confident in every aspect of my life. I'm confident with women, have lots of chat, and love being in crowds. I relish public speaking. I'm very sporty and almost too confident in some ways. I never shy away from ANYTHING. Ever. I'm open to trying anything once. If it's new, dangerous, a buzz, or just plain stupid, I'm up for it. This hasn't always worked in my favour, I must admit. As you know by now, I worked as a dancer/entertainer/male stripper for sixteen years and had no qualms about getting naked for just about anyone, if they shoved a few hundred quid in front of my face. In fact, I'd take my clothes off at every opportunity given half the chance.

BUT, 16 years in and out of pubs and clubs all over Europe at least five times per week damaged my hearing a little. Mixed with the fact that my mum is hard of hearing, I now wear two hearing aids that I really fucking hate, if I'm honest with you. At times, I've been embarrassed when I've noticed someone spot them. I've purposely not turned my head at times when I've wanted and despite all my friends saying it's nothing, to me at times it's made me feel like I have a disability.

I've often felt like there was something wrong with me and that I wasn't good enough. It's made me feel very uncomfortable. Sounds stupid, right? Maybe you can relate in some way? It's taken me years to get comfortable with this in my head and I'd get annoyed at myself for letting it bother me, but it has, there's no denying that. This is something I never thought I would write. A few years ago, I would have been too embarrassed to admit this failure to anyone, never mind writing it in a book for all and sundry.

The truth is, without my hearing aids, I would miss a lot and even with them I have to concentrate on what you're saying. I'd pay any amount of money to fix this situation, but now, there isn't anything that can be done. Admittedly, there are a few bonuses. I have a disabled rail card, which has saved me a fortune in rail travel over the last few years and the look on the conductors' faces as they check my ticket is just priceless. And with the amount of rubbish a lot of people spout these days, it's not a bad thing that I miss half of it. So there, that's out in the open. I feel better having said that – ish. That's my secret. Maybe I should send you some cash as by writing this for you to read I feel like I've seen a counsellor now.

You might be thinking, "If that's all Gav has to worry about then he is in a pretty fortunate position". Maybe I am. Maybe I'm just being silly, but to me it's felt monumental at times. So, what's this got to do with you? Well, you've got a few insecurities, haven't you? Ones that hold you back. Ones that you know are silly but feel huge inside your head. I know what it's like taking that first step. Maybe you know you should do something about your current situation, but you're scared to take the first step. Maybe you've "failed" before and don't want to waste your time failing again. Maybe you've been told you can never lose weight because you're "big boned".

How do I know you've got insecurities in your head? Because everyone I've ever worked with has. Even the most successful person in the world has insecurities. Every human on the planet has. It's embarrassing, a little awkward at times and some of you really WILL be stepping out of your comfort zone. Making any change in a big part of your life is uncomfortable; especially when it comes to excess weight you may have accumulated over the last few years. I'm telling you to face your fear head on and the only way to do that is to make a move. Take that first step, however uncomfortable.

What's your secret? I've shown you mine. How about you show me yours?

Go ahead and write down your number one fear or insecurity below. Don't worry; no one else will see this. Be honest with yourself. This fear may be holding you back and usually it's not even real.

My no. 1 fear is:

_____

10. CREATING A PLAN

"To achieve great things, two things are needed: a plan and not quite enough time"

- Leonard Bernstein -

One size does not fit all when it comes to creating a plan. Much like a human fingerprint, everyone is unique in that everyone has a different goal that is relevant for him or her. Weight loss may be one person's goal, but for someone else, overcoming a serious health challenge may be the main priority. Everyone has different genetics and a different starting point. Someone may be very experienced or a complete beginner. Everyone has different capabilities, motivations, and degrees of desire to change. All these points and more should be taken into consideration, and your plan should reflect this.

Whatever your experience or life situation, your plan must be sustainable, manageable, and you need to be consistent in following it. There's no point creating a plan for you that you can't commit to. Very often I see people at the beginning of the new year saying, "I want to lose weight". They commit themselves to going to the gym five days a week. From experience, this person will most likely fail and fail fast because going from zero to five times a week is not sustainable for most people. When I work with a client, if they haven't moved for several years, I will ask them, "what exercise do you like to do and how many 30-minute sessions can you commit to every week?"

"I like to jog, and I can commit to that three times per week".

"How will you ensure you stick to that?" I ask. "I'll go with a friend of mine who runs every week and I just know I will run two more times".

When a client says it, it becomes their truth. I'm not telling them to do anything. They tell me. That's the beauty of coaching. What do you like? What can you commit to? That's your truth.

Is jogging the best activity for weight loss? Possibly not. But telling a client who has done nothing for years that weight training is the best way to burn body fat, though it's factually correct, is not always the best step. 3 x 30 minutes per week for the first three or four weeks is a great start. Now we have some momentum. This takes the client up to twelve sessions in a month. That's way more powerful than doing five in the first week and then nothing in the second week because they're burnt out and can't commit to it, or even worse, they get injured. Consistency and sustainability are the keys here. Getting those three sessions in over a seven-day period. That's usually all it takes to get results for someone starting from the couch.

There's no strict schedule and this allows for life to get in the way. A plan that demands too much too soon is destined to fail. Imagine a five-day per week programme and in week one, you only manage to do three sessions. This can be the kiss of death for many clients. "I've failed again. I can't even complete week one. I'm such a loser". I've seen it happen. The client quits in week two. Disappears like a virgin on prom night. Gone forever.

Your busy work, family, and life commitments won't change. It's your life. So, we work the plan around those commitments, not the other way around. If you don't follow the plan, you're not on the right plan for you. Your plan should be achievable, even with the toughest of schedules.

Kenny worked with me last year and struggled with the exercise element of his programme. His incredibly busy schedule and love of all things food and wine, although not excuses, left us with some work to do.

Here's what Kenny had to say:

"As I type I have completed Gav's twelve-week programme - I have made tremendous progress with my weight loss goals by loosing 12kgs of weight, five and a half inches off my waist line but not just that - working with him has given me a different perspective on life. I was skeptical initially - how could someone working with you from a distance really have impact? We had a very open and frank initial call, which lasted about an hour but during that time he had captured

enough information to build a programme. I am a lover of food, dining out and my glasses of wine but rather than ruling everything out all the time, Gav made practical recommendations on how I could minimise, choose more wisely and sometimes cut out.

The simple but effective model of watching the calories, understanding the calories and how you could be smarter with what and when you are eating made a considerable difference. It also takes account of the fact that you must live and work, there will always be events - you can still live your normal life but in a smarter, more calorie efficient manner.

Throughout the weekly calls he gets you to complete exercises that 1) cause you to dig deep into your life and 2) without any commentary from him cause you to reflect on what's important and what adjustments are needed.

I believe that anyone who struggles with the rollercoaster of weight management as I have can only benefit from engaging with and being coached by Gav".

The "Small Wins" Philosophy

Did you do some type of movement today? Did you sweat? Did you eat three meals that were high in protein? Did you drink two litres of water? Are you going to get to sleep on time?

Many people are looking for the "big secret" to success, but there really is no secret. Small daily wins over time will lead to big results in anything you do in life. These tiny successes might seem innocuous but consistent, daily action on the basics leads to fantastic results. That's the "big secret". The truth is, you all have the ability and the capability to achieve better results than you can ever imagine if you'd only look at this from the right perspective.

"Say it ain't so Gav, this can't be the truth". Well my friends, I'm happy to say it is. It's like compound interest. You start saving a little each month. In the first few years, not much happens. With consistent saving, month after month, year after year, the magic starts to happen. In 20 years, you've accrued a fortune. This is the same with your health and weight loss. The good news is that it's not going to take 20 years to get you to your goal, but it will take consistent, daily action.

The Japanese word 'kaizen' means ongoing improvement. In business, it refers to activities that continuously improve all functions and involve all employees from the CEO to the assembly line workers. Adopting a 'kaizen' philosophy to your health could be a great idea. Select the area of life you want to improve. In this case, it's your health. Identify small, specific tasks that will contribute to your goal (small daily wins). Prioritise your tasks and actions (nutrition and exercise) and create a timeline (set your goal with a date/deadline). Track your progress (weight, measurements, pictures and performance) and continue until you reach your goal (desired outcome).

I know there are some of you who'll be reading this and think, "it's very hard for me to stick to a plan because of my travel schedule, my commitments, and one week never seems to be the same as the last". I get it. I understand that for many, this is your life, but let's reframe this whole deal shall we? If your plans get disrupted with life, then how about being grateful that you have the means to even go to the gym at all? How about being grateful that your life is busy because there are many people on this planet that have nothing; and I mean nothing. No food, water, shoes on their feet or a place to sleep. Puts things into perspective doesn't it? With this in mind, missing a workout doesn't seem so important does it? I know it's all relative, but still.

Big "MO"

I'd been thinking and toying with the idea of writing a book for about two years. It wasn't this book funnily enough; it wasn't any book in particular. It was just a book. I knew I wanted to write one. Probably a little bit of ego mixed with the fact I love reading and writing. OK, no probably about it, it was definitely ego. I'd start and then stop. Write 1,000 words of something, but with no real direction. I told a few people I was writing a book, but I didn't even know what the book was about. It was a mess to be honest. It was my mess and I was proud of it, but a bunch of words on a laptop won't change the world. I needed help.

My good friend, Rachel Holmes AKA "The Cap'n", an accomplished and published author herself said, "Just get your pen out, or your laptop, and write. Get up and write whether you feel like it or not". She said, "It doesn't matter what you write. Just write". These were the smartest words ever said to me and I want to thank you Rachel for imparting your words of wisdom onto me. I now have the pleasure of passing that wisdom onto you guys.

Some days you will wake up and just won't feel motivated. Regardless of whether you feel motivated or not, starting with something small can lead to something very big. You've moved the needle in the right direction, perhaps only a touch, but towards your goal. Like writing a paragraph of words in a book, a walk around the block is progress. A walk around the block leads to you eating a healthy breakfast. It's a start. Big "Mo" kicks in. You now have momentum. It's a small win and we all know what happens with small wins don't we?

Once you do one thing, the rest becomes a lot easier. You build that mental fortitude. You see the positive action that you've taken, and the grit needed, and you've created a neural pathway in your brain. The success groove becomes deeper and stronger, and your desire in turn strengthens to repeat this action. You acknowledge that small success and it's like a "boot up the proverbial". It sends a message to you that "I can do this. I don't have to be perfect and I'm a long way from achieving my goal - but I know I can get there".

11. WHAT YOU MUST KNOW

"Knowledge is a treasure, but practice is the key to it"

- Lao Tzu -

There's no magical silver bullet. There is no quantum leap from A to Z. Results take time and they require hard work. Many clients that work with me have spent years neglecting their diet, not exercising, and yet expect miracles in just weeks. I had one client that wanted to lose four stone in 12 weeks. "I'm fucking good but I'm not David Blaine", I said. They've taken years to get out of shape, and although it won't take the same time to change, it'll take some time, patience, and consistent effort. Small changes over time lead to massive results. Have I said that before?

Nutrition

I often get clients asking me the same thing repeatedly when they see someone else getting amazing results. Questions like, "what are they doing that I'm not? What are you telling them that you haven't told me?". The answer is absolutely nothing. They're getting results because they're doing the boring, mundane activities like tracking their calories, keeping an eye on their protein levels and exercising consistently. And they have patience.

It's not sexy, it's not the "in thing" that half of Hollywood are doing. It's the basics, every day, with consistency. That's the key to a radical and long - lasting shift in your health and weight loss. I wish it wasn't true. I wish I had something better for you, something sexier, but I don't. If you want to know the truth, then read on. If this doesn't sound like your brand of vodka, I suggest you stop reading this book now.

Nutrition is more important than exercise when it comes to losing weight and getting in shape. If you're reading this book and you've got weight to lose, you're eating more calories than you need to. It's that simple. To lose fat you're going to have to burn more energy than the number of calories you take in. Here endeth the lesson. OK - there's a little more to it than that. We will look at the calories that will make a difference to how you function, but for now; let's take it back to the basics of what you need to know.

Just What is a Calorie?

A calorie is the amount of heat needed to raise the temperature of one gram of water by one degree Celsius. Calories in food provide energy in the form of heat that fuels our body. Our body stores and "burns" calories as fuel. A calorie isn't actually a thing. It's simply a unit of measurement of energy. Everything we do relies on the energy that fuels it, and that energy is measured in calories.

One gram of protein and one gram of carbohydrates each contain four calories, while one gram of fat has nine calories. One gram of alcohol has seven. When we know that, we can work out how many calories or how much energy a food source or meal contains. This is important. On a fundamental level, if you consume too many calories you will gain weight. Excess calories not used for energy are stored as body fat.

How Many Calories Do You Need?

The NHS suggest that the average woman needs 2000kcal per day and the average man needs 2500kcal per day to maintain their body weight. This is far too simplistic in my opinion. What does average mean? Everyone's needs are different but working it out for yourself can be as simple as knowing what you do in your day-to-day life. If you're tall with a large build and you exercise frequently, you will need more calories than someone who is smaller and leads a sedentary life. Height, weight, gender, age, and activity level all play a big role in your caloric needs.

Your BMR or Basal Metabolic Rate; the number of calories you need to perform basic metabolic functions and daily physical activities is the number of calories you need to eat to maintain your weight. You can use various formulae designed by scientists or you can get tested in a lab, to find out exactly how many calories you need. Alternatively keep reading to find out the formula I use with all my clients that is super simple, but extremely effective.

You may have heard the term "macronutrient". The three main macronutrients are carbohydrate, protein, and fat. Macro means above one gram, and micro means below one gram. When someone says, "what are your macros, bro?" they are referring to the ratio of carbohydrates, protein, and fat in your diet.

Carbohydrates

There are complex carbs and simple carbs. Complex carbs are things like peas, beans, certain fruits, whole grains, and vegetables. Simple carbs are naturally found in fruits, milk, and in processed and refined foods like sweets, chocolate, syrups, table sugar, and soft drinks. When we eat carbohydrates, the body breaks them down to produce energy. The body can use protein and fat for energy, but the easiest fuel for our body to use is carbohydrate. Carbs taste great too, so be very wary of anybody that says to cut carbs from your diet if you're trying to lose weight.

Carbohydrates have been given a bad rap over the years and I think unfairly so. The primary source of fuel for the brain is glucose, which comes from carbohydrate. If you want to function at work with some type of efficiency, don't eliminate carbs from your diet entirely. Cutting carbs from your diet may produce weight loss but it's a reduction in calories that made you lose weight, not the reduction in carbs.

Best Sources of Carbs

It's probably wise to avoid eating too many processed carbohydrates like sugar, cakes, biscuits, and sweets. They're laden with calories, nutrient deficient, and tend to score very high on the glycemic index. The glycemic index is a guide to show the speed at which a food source is broken down and raises blood sugar. Pure glucose is rated at 100. Food sources that rank high on the "GI" will give you an immediate energy boost by raising your blood sugar, but often this is accompanied with an insulin spike and a crash in energy. This could affect your food choices for the rest of the day. We will look at this in more detail in the chapter on insulin and hormones. Better choices could consist of carbs that are lower on the "GI" and score

55 or below out of a possible 100, such as oatmeal, some fruits, pumpernickel bread, lentils, and sweet potato, to name a few. Knowing the "GI" of certain foods is important and may come in handy to a certain extent but don't get too wrapped up in that. Later in the book I will show you that insulin isn't the be all and end all when it comes to losing body fat.

For your reference, go to **www.theghgmethod.com/bonus** for a printable "GI" to check all your favourite foods.

Protein

The word protein is derived from the Greek word "proteios" meaning primary or most important. The Greeks had it right. Protein is an important component of every cell in the body. Your body uses protein to build and repair tissues, bones, muscles, skin, blood, and every other substance in your body. Protein is made up of 20 amino acids, nine of which are essential, and we need to obtain from food. They can't be synthesized or created by your body. Animals and fish contain all the essential amino acids and are called "complete proteins". Plants also contain proteins, but they're referred to as "incomplete proteins". Vegetarians & vegans must be smart by mixing and matching their food sources to obtain adequate sources of "complete" proteins.

Best Sources of Protein

Animal proteins such as beef, chicken, turkey, fish, and eggs contain the best sources of complete protein. More exotic meats such as elk, buffalo, ostrich, kangaroo, and wild boar are also fantastic sources of complete protein and tend to be very lean, while often containing a valuable source of omega-3 fatty acids. Whatever meat you decide to go for, always opt for free-range or grass-fed if you can. This means the animals have been allowed to graze in their natural habitat and have eaten grass, which they are designed to eat in the wild.

Most of the protein we consume tends to be from factory-farmed animals that have been pumped full of steroids and other artificial hormones for accelerated growth and disease prevention. This is great for the farmer and the meat industry but not so great for us, the consumer. Free-range and grass-fed will give you much more clout when it comes to nutrition and you won't be consuming the potentially harmful cocktail of chemicals used in today's farming industries.

Eggs are one of the most complete protein sources on the planet, rich in nutrients and essential fats. In my opinion, they definitely constitute a "superfood". Not all eggs are the same. Poorly kept, battery-farmed chickens produce horrendous eggs. You really do get what you pay for with eggs (and life in general). Buy 24 eggs for a quid from your local corner store and you can guess the quality of the eggs. Choose free-range, organic eggs whenever possible. You will pay a lot more, but the egg will have a better vitamin and mineral profile, and much more omega-3 fatty acids. Omega-3's are essential for our health and aptly come under the title of EFAs, which is short for essential fatty acids. See the section on fish oil and omega-3s for a more detailed look at why we need them.

Protein is often seen as the magical macronutrient when it comes to weight loss. This is for several reasons. It's highly satiating, which means it keeps you feeling fuller for longer. I sound like a leading supermarket. Yes, Sainsbury's have it right by naming a range of high protein meals "fuller for longer". In many ways, it's an appetite suppressant. Secondly, protein will help to build or at least maintain lean body mass (LBM). Muscle tissue is your body's fat burning machinery. The more you have, the more calories you burn, just by existing. Muscle tissue is very expensive to maintain metabolically, which means that someone with more muscle will burn more calories when just sitting, walking, and even sleeping, than the person with less muscle. Therefore, a more muscular man can tend to eat more than a man with less muscle and not store excess body fat. Thirdly, protein has a high "TEF". TEF - the "thermic effect of food" is the amount of energy required to digest and process the food you eat. Also called thermogenesis, it accounts for approximately 10% of your total daily energy expenditure.

Protein is the most thermogenic macronutrient. Although certain foods can affect your metabolism, there are no specific fat burning foods, and ultimately, it's calories alone that will determine if you gain or lose weight. With protein being more than double the thermic rate of carbs, you can see why I suggest your diet should be high in protein.

Your protein intake will cause the body to release important neurotransmitters. These are chemical messengers that transmit signals to the brain. Dopamine, which is made from the amino acid tyrosine; found in chicken, turkey, and fish among other things, is one of them. Dopamine is a key factor in motivation, productivity, and focus. It can boost drive and confidence and is associated with high-octane pursuits like adrenalin-based sports or being in love. Stimuli such as food, sex, and cocaine reinforce the dopamine reward pathway. Becoming addicted to high protein meals as opposed to sex and cocaine will only enhance your quest for fat loss and optimal health, but of course, the choice is yours.

There is one big thing that affects your metabolism that can't go unmentioned. Genetics. Some people just have a much faster metabolism than others. Some people can process carbohydrates far better then others and seem to be able to eat whatever they want, without storing body fat. All the calories we eat will either be used as energy or stored as fat. This is called "nutrient partitioning". If you're a good nutrient partitioner, all the calories you eat will go to building muscle and all the calories you store as fat are used efficiently for energy.

Do you know someone that is really built, with granite like pecs and chiseled abs, yet they don't even train that much? We all know one or two of them, don't we? The bastards. If you are one of "them", you don't need this book. If you haven't been gifted with godlike genes that would make Achilles himself green with envy, and are merely mortal, my advice for you is simple. Choose better parents next time round.

You might be thinking, "Well, if I eat a diet that contains a ton of high protein and highly thermogenic foods, I can lose weight. Sounds great!" But it's not as simple as that. You can see why it's extremely important for your health as well as for your fat loss, but let's not get confused here. One gram of protein still has 4kcal, which is the same as one gram of carbohydrate. It still contains energy and if too many calories are consumed, regardless of the source, you will store fat. That said, a good quality source of protein with most meals is considered a smart move if fat loss and body composition is important to you.

Whilst we are on the subject of protein, I often get asked how much do we need daily, and can you eat too much? The RDA (recommended daily amount) is 0.8g/kg of bodyweight, per day. This equates to about 60 grams per day if you weigh 75kg. This is to ensure basic recovery, enzyme synthesis and muscle repair, along with all the other functions in the body that require it. For *optimal* performance and fat loss however, the picture is very different.

At the beginning of this book, I said that you wouldn't find study after study and references galore in this book. I didn't tell you the entire truth. Here's one:

A study from Jose Antonio et al. on "Protein & Exercise" was published in JISSN (Journal International Society of Sports Nutrition) on 26th September 2007. The results showed that 1.4-2g/kg/day was a good range for exercising individuals and concluded with, **"No substantive evidence that protein intakes in the ranges suggested above will have adverse effects in healthy, exercising individuals".**

What this means is that for example, if you weigh 80kg and are exercising, you could have as much as 160g of protein per day without any negative consequences. Later in this chapter I will go into exactly how much you need and why, and I'll explain the formula I use with all my clients.

Bodybuilders, powerlifters, and "strongman" competitors have been known to take much higher amounts of protein with no adverse effects but for most of you reading this book, it's probably not relevant. The truth is, you will probably be bored of eating protein long before you have any cause for concern. A small side note: please don't get your nutritional advice from the newspapers. They are usually misinformed and the information they print is often inaccurate. There are currently no valid studies that link protein intake with cancer, nor will it harm your kidneys, unless you have a problem with your kidneys already.

Fat

To start with, why is fat called fat? It's very confusing for many people. Have you ever thought twice about eating dietary fat because it will be stored as fat on the body? I'm sure you have, but the good news is it doesn't work like that. Fat contains 9kcal per gram, making it over twice as calorific as carbs or protein, but as I mentioned before, too many calories make you fat, not the consumption of an important macronutrient. Dietary fat has absolutely nothing to do with stored body fat. Fat is an important and vital part of your diet.

There are three types of fat. Saturated fat: usually in animal fats, red meat, and cheese. Monounsaturated fats, which are in vegetables, nuts, seeds, fish, avocado and olive oil. Finally, polyunsaturated fats: these can be broken down into two further categories: omega-3 and omega-6. Both are essential and beneficial to your health but there tends to be an over consumption of omega-6 in the western diet from sources such as factory farmed poultry and eggs, vegetable oils and of course, processed foods.

It's important to get a good ratio between them. Current studies suggest that many people have a ratio of 16:1 in favour of omega-6s due to the food sources we eat containing a lot more omega-6s, and less and less omega-3s. Evidence has suggested that the ratio should be somewhere between 4:1

and 2:1, which means we need a lot less omega-6 and a lot more omega-3 in our diet. "Why?", I hear you ask? Well basically, omega-6 is pro-inflammatory and omega-3 is anti-inflammatory.

Inflammation is essential for survival because it protects your body from infection and injury. But too much inflammation can contribute to degenerative diseases such as heart disease, arthritis, Alzheimer's, diabetes, and various types of cancer. There are multiple omega-3s but the most important ones are EPA (eicosapentaenoic acid) and DHA (docosahexaenoic acid), primarily found in fatty fish, seafood, and fish oil, and alpha-linolenic acid primarily found in high plant foods such as flax seed, chia seeds, and walnuts. (No, I can't pronounce them either).

The best sources of omega-3 are in fish such as salmon, sardines, mackerel and anchovies. You may have experienced your parents or grandparents telling you to have a cod liver oil tablet as a kid. Sometimes the old wisdom still rings true. Your grandmother was talking some sense. Although things have moved on from there, she was essentially telling you to have a cod liver oil tablet because it was good "brain food". They're called essential fatty acids for a reason. They're essential for health with many benefits that have been proven. Fish oil has been shown to reduce inflammation and soreness after a workout. It can lubricate the joints and aid in the prevention of arthritis and osteoporosis, and has been shown to reduce symptoms of depression, as well as acting as a mood enhancer. (See the chapter on supplements for more on information on this). Quality is paramount with fish oil. Always buy a brand that is reputable and has been tested for - and purified of - heavy metals like mercury and lead.

Tracking Calories

I often get clients saying, "I don't want to track my calories: it's boring, hard work, and too time consuming". If that was true (which it isn't), it's a bloody lot easier than being 30lbs or more overweight and hating how you look and feel. You decide. You choose your variety of hard work. Some people can reduce their calories by guesswork, and you know what? If it works then that's great. If that person can lose the weight they want and maintain it by guesswork, I say go for it. In fact, if you can get to that stage when you don't have to track your calories, that's the aim. For most people in the beginning, that just isn't a reality. To those people and maybe you reading this – track your damn calories. It's the only effective way of knowing what is going on.

There are many apps available to track calories. I like to use MyFitnessPal. It's easy to use and very easy to teach clients how to use. Download the app MyFitnessPal on your phone and upgrade to premium. Here you can very easily log your food and calories. There's a barcode scanner to make it simple. It takes literally two minutes after each meal to record or scan what you've just eaten.

Calorie Deficit, Calorie Surplus and Maintenance

The act of losing body fat or weight is actually very simple but not necessarily easy. If it were, everyone would be at his or her ideal weight. The mechanics of weight loss are very simple. (The mindset is not so simple). If you burn more calories than you consume, this is what's called being in a "calorie deficit." Ultimately, this is our aim. In fact, it's the only way to lose body fat. If you consume more calories than you burn, you're in what's called a "calorie surplus". You'll gain weight in either body fat or muscle, or both, but usually body fat. Eating the number of calories so you neither gain nor lose weight, staying the same, is called "maintenance". Our aim is to be in what I call "the sweet spot". This is where you're burning more calories than you consume and are just in a deficit, but not so much that you're ravenously hungry. When you get this right, you can lose body fat and still feel good, and have high energy levels.

A word of warning: if you drop your calories too low and create a large deficit, you will lose weight fast. Some fat for sure, but mostly the weight will come from lean body mass. This is the kiss of death for your weight loss journey. Muscle or lean body mass is our fat burning machinery. You'll burn more calories and lose body fat, just by having it on your skeleton. Our aim is to, at minimum, preserve all the muscle you have, and in some cases increase the muscle you have - and burn the excess body fat.

Someone says, "I know a friend that ate 800 calories every day for four weeks and lost 20 pounds". Yes, this may be true, but what a horrendous four weeks. Deprivation, pain, hunger, and generally feeling shitty about life. It's not the way; it's not sustainable, not fun and is just plain stupid. The best diet in the world is the one you can stay on the longest. In fact, it's not a diet; it's a lifestyle. A healthy way of eating with no start or end point. It's just how you eat.

Every diet on the market is designed to do one thing and one thing only. Create a calorie deficit. Here are some of the popular diets on the market today: the paleo diet, the Cambridge diet, the carnivore diet, the vegan diet, the South Beach diet, the cabbage soup diet, intermittent fasting, the ketogenic diet, the low fat, high carb diet, the high fat, low carb diet, the high protein, low carb diet. The list goes on and on. These are just a few that came to mind as I wrote this chapter. Any one of these diets will yield weight loss results if the user is in a calorie deficit and persistent in following it. Some of these diets have some sense attached to them. I'm not going to beat around the bush here: others are just plain fucking stupid and, in some cases, quite dangerous.

The "2-1-1" Fat Loss Formula

It's tried and tested with hundreds of clients and I use it personally myself. Welcome to the "2-1-1" fat loss formula, which originally came from my friend and nutritionist Matt Lovell. He told me about it about seven years ago. Matt was the nutritionist who helped the England Rugby squad win the World Cup back in 2003 and currently works with many Olympic gold medalists in athletics and Premiership winning football teams. It's safe to say he knows his onions. I realised I had been using something similar myself naturally with clients, but I hadn't put a name to it.

Go to **www.theghgmethod.com/bonus** to download and find out exactly how the 2-1-1 fat loss formula works. Go there now and come back.

You back here? Good.

Here's the important bit - you only need to worry about two numbers: hitting your protein goal and your total calorie goal. I like my clients to hit their protein. If they do that and don't exceed their total calories it doesn't really matter how they make up the rest. It's largely irrelevant. Carbs and fat are just sources of fuel. Don't worry if you're over one and under the other some days, just hit your protein goal and calorie goal, and you'll be on track. If you start to lose weight, we know it's working. If you're not losing weight, we may need to look at the macros a little closer.

This formula allows the client a lot of flexibility in their diet. I want you to look at your calories as a balancing act. Take your daily calories, for example; say 1,500kcal a day, and times it by seven for seven days in the week. This equates to 10,500kcal over the week. If you were eating 1,500kcal per day and your protein levels are high, you're losing weight, guess what? You're in the "sweet spot". You can now start to have fun with this. It doesn't matter how or when you eat those calories. You could eat 3,000kcal one day and then nothing the next. The result and subsequent fat loss would be the same. You could miss breakfast and lunch and eat all 1500kcal for dinner. The resulting fat loss, if you are in a calorie deficit will be the same.

I'm not suggesting you do that, but you could. If you know you have a birthday meal or something similar and it's going to be large, here's a great tip for you: under eat during the day. Have a small breakfast and small lunch, allowing 1,000 calories or more to play with for dinner. It really doesn't matter when or how you get these calories. What matters is the total number of calories over the day and the week.

The food sources you choose will help you adhere to your overall calorie intake. A massive bowl of Frosties and a glass of OJ at 7am may have you tearing your packed lunch open at 10am. The chances of you overeating are higher than if you had scrambled eggs and avocado. This is all down to various hormones like insulin, leptin and ghrelin. I will address these in chapter 14. But if you hit your calories, at the end of the day it doesn't matter.

I often get asked, "can you lose fat eating crap calories?" The truth is, yes you can, if you are in a calorie deficit. Is it advisable? Well think about this. Every cell in your body is made from the food you consume. Food isn't just food. Food is information. Every single molecule of food you eat can impact your genetic expression and has a huge impact on your hormonal profile and DNA expression. It will affect how you show up in the world with your energy, your thoughts, and your mood. You literally have the power to help your body create the best version of you and potentially avoid many degenerative diseases. It all starts with the food you eat. Genetic predisposition is an increased likelihood of developing a particular disease based on a person's genetic makeup. This doesn't mean you will get the disease but the choices you make in your lifestyle from things like food, alcohol, drugs, and sleep all play a huge role. Genetics load the gun and lifestyle pulls the trigger.

That said, if eating a little bit of what you like each day helps you adhere to your diet and keeps you in a calorie deficit for longer, that can only be a good thing. I like to eat as healthily as I can most of the time because I know I'm made from the food choices I make. I have a few meals at the weekend where I go off-piste and enjoy myself, but I bring it back under control on a Monday. I just perform much better this way, and I think you will too. I love this quote from Alan Aragon, "every meal is a short-term investment in how you feel and perform, a mid-term investment in how you look, and a long-term investment in your freedom from disease".

Constructing your diet

When constructing a diet plan, there are a few rules that I like to adhere to. Go to **www.theghgmethod.com/bonus** to download my "Diet Rules Checklist" and a few sample menus that you may find useful.

Now some of you will be thinking, "How can I track things accurately if I eat at the office canteen or buy a load of meat from the butcher?" It's a good question that is often asked. You will never be able to track perfectly and that's OK. No one is perfect. Everyone that uses MyFitnessPal, or any tracker like this, will rely on a certain amount of guesswork. It will never be perfect. Over time, with practice, you'll get better and better at estimating the portions you have on your plate.

If it really means that much to you in terms of losing body fat, perhaps you won't always go to the canteen. Maybe it might be better to buy something from Marks & Spencer's, or Sainsbury's, or Tesco's, or whatever is nearest to you, instead of the canteen. Better still, you might want to prep your own food where you know exactly what you're eating. I understand that this is not always going to be possible for some people, but if this one meal at lunchtime in the staff canteen was affecting your weight loss, it might be wise to look at an alternative.

I was coaching a client recently called Bob. His situation was not unlike many of you. Busy with commitments from work, family, and life. When we started working together, he wouldn't even download the app on his phone. "I don't have time for crap like this" – his words. OK, no problem. I asked him if he had lost any weight. He said no. I said to him, "do you want to lose weight?" He said, "of course I do, that's why I paid you". Bob was a bit rude at times, but I knew that this was just a defence mechanism. He was embarrassed about his weight and even though he had reached out for help, he was using classic deflection tactics with me. We arranged a one-to-one consultation. I told him in no uncertain terms that using the app was crucial to him getting results. I explained that given his circumstances, he was very unlikely to achieve anything if he didn't track his calories. He reluctantly listened and took on board what I was saying. Long story short, Bob went on to drop 8kg in his final six weeks of working with me. In the first six weeks, he didn't lose a single pound.

Bob's testimonial:

"I was extremely skeptical of Gav's advice when I first started

working with him but after a pretty stern conversation with him, I eventually came to realise that I probably should follow his advice. I must admit; his coaching was brilliant, and I was happy with losing 8kg in just 6 weeks".

Supplements

There are many supplements available on the market today. Some are credible. Some work and do what they're intended to do, but many have no evidence to back up their proposed efficacy, despite their claims. Unfortunately, this doesn't stop the industry growing year after year into a multi-billion pound industry. Over the years I have tried many. I've been happy to be a guinea pig and to be honest; it's hard to know what works and what doesn't. Many times, I've wanted to believe a certain product has worked and is helping me, but I have no real evidence to confirm that.

Over the years of working in the industry, I now only recommend a few key supplements and products that I believe to work, as suggested by the evidence and literature, as well as my own experience. The truth is, many people would get much better results from simply cleaning up their diet, addressing their sleep issues, and moving more. In my opinion, that would radically change how most people operate in their day. Once the basics are covered, supplements enhance an already solid baseline level of exercise and diet habits and practices.

Here are my top 5 supplements you might consider using yourself:

1. Whey protein - All dairy (milk) products contain whey, one of the main proteins in dairy. During processing into a powder, the liquid milk is separated into solid curds (casein) and liquid (the whey). Whey protein is a complete protein, meaning it contains all the essential amino acids your body needs (i.e. can't produce on its own and is thus needed from food sources) to continue protein synthesis aka: building muscle.

A common misconception about whey protein is that is contains special muscle building properties that make you sprout huge muscles. Whey protein is purely used to increase the amount of protein in an individual's diet if they can't obtain enough whole protein from their food. It's sometimes easier to mix up a protein shake at your desk than to have a chicken breast in a container. It's quick, convenient, and may be cost effective for many. I recommend a client use whey protein only if they struggle to get enough protein from food; not to use it instead of eating a proper meal.

2. Multi-vitamin and mineral complex - There are 13 essential vitamins and 16 essential minerals that we should be able to obtain from our diet. These are largely responsible for protection against nutritional deficiencies, improving energy and performance, and disease prevention. Athletes and people with a physically active lifestyle need more nutrients than the average non-active person to support muscle recovery and any fitness related goal. Strenuous exercise is also associated with oxidative stress and tissue damage, so athletes require a higher intake of antioxidant nutrients such as vitamins C and E.

The evidence is mixed when it comes to whether we need to supplement multi-vitamins. Some experts believe we can get all the nutrients we need from a "balanced diet". Other experts believe that even with a balanced diet, levels of nutrients are far from adequate when it comes to optimal health.

The truth is, many people don't even hit their RDA (recommended daily amount) levels. Several large-scale observational studies show that many people simply don't achieve nutritional sufficiency through diet alone. This may be caused partly by declining soil quality, which means fresh fruit and vegetables aren't as nutritious as they were 70 years ago. This coupled with the fact that chemicals in the air, food, and water provide an unprecedented toxic load that we are exposed to daily. For this reason alone, my foot is firmly in the camp of supplementation.

Composition and quality can vary from product to product so choose a high-quality brand that has been tested and guaranteed for potency. A quality brand will ensure that the nutrients will be provided in their most bioavailable form to enhance digestion and absorption.

3. Fish oil - One of the most popular supplements on the market today and widely researched. It has been shown to improve many of the risk factors of heart attacks, such as high cholesterol, blood pressure, and triglycerides. Studies have shown that fish oil supplementation can prevent the onset, or improve the symptoms, of some mental disorders like schizophrenia and bipolar and prevent symptoms of mental decline. Fish oil has strong anti-inflammatory effects and can help reduce symptoms of inflammatory diseases, especially rheumatoid arthritis. Your skin can become damaged by too much sun exposure or by natural ageing. Fish oil may help maintain healthy skin and prevent skin disorders such as psoriasis and dermatitis. Supplementation in pregnant and breastfeeding women may improve both hand and eye coordination in infants, improve visual development, and help reduce the risk of allergies. The list goes on.

If you are not eating oily fish 2-3 times per week, you will probably benefit from supplementing with high quality fish oil.

4. Vitamin D - It's sometimes called the "sunshine vitamin" because your body produces vitamin D naturally when it's exposed to direct sunlight. As a vitamin and hormone, it stands alone amongst its peers and plays a pivotal role in cell metabolism, cardiac health, immune function, neurological support, and systemic inflammation, which is the process central to the onset of many chronic diseases.

Vitamin D may play a role in decreasing your risk of multiple sclerosis, decreasing your risk of heart disease, and reduce your likelihood of getting the flu. Research has shown that vitamin D might play an important role in regulating mood and warding off depression. Many factors can affect your ability to get sufficient amounts of vitamin D through the sun alone, such as being in an area with high pollution like a city environment, using sunscreen, and having darker skin. People with darker skin have higher levels of melanin making it harder for the skin to absorb vitamin D. Only a few foods contain vitamin D naturally such as salmon, sardines, and egg yolks; while just 15-30 minutes of full-body exposure to sunlight is enough to provide all the vitamin D the body needs. However, it's often difficult to obtain this even in sunny climates. For this reason, many people are chronically deficient in vitamin D.

In my opinion, it is essential to supplement with a minimum of 2000-3000 IU of vitamin D per day.

5. Creatine - Creatine is found naturally in our diet when we consume meat and fish. The body also produces it internally, but it is excreted daily, which is why many people supplement it. Creatine is one of the most researched supplements and has produced many studies to prove its efficacy. It's a natural supplement used to boost athletic performance. It's not only safe; it's one of the most popular supplements and most effective in building muscle and strength. It can increase your muscles' phosphocreatine stores, which help with the formation of new ATP, the key molecule your cells use for energy, and all basic functions of life. It helps your cells produce more energy, which improves high intensity performance. It has also been shown to help with muscular endurance, muscle fatigue, recovery, and even brain performance.

3-5 grams taken daily has been proven to be the optimal dose for maximum athletic benefits.

Go to **www.theghgmethod.com/bonus** to download a checklist of what to look for in the supplements you buy and the brands that I personally use and recommend, along with a few other notable supplements you might want to look at.

Exercise

Weight Training: Compound vs Isolation Exercises

Compound exercises are multi-joint movements that work several muscles or muscle groups at once. A classic example of this would be a squat or bench press. An isolation exercise is a movement that isolates one muscle group only. An example of this would be a bicep curl or a calf raise.

Compound movements create the greatest changes in body composition in the shortest time because multiple joints are being used at once, meaning more weight can be used. They recruit much more muscle mass, which in turn uses more calories. Compound movements get the most "bang for your buck", so to speak, and when it comes to building lean muscle mass and losing weight, you can't beat them. There is a time and a place for isolation exercises but to be honest, if weight loss is your goal, then you can forget about isolation exercises until you can see your six-pack.

Lean body mass is the name of the game here. Muscle is your body's fat burning machinery. The more lean muscle tissue you can build or at least maintain, the faster and easier you can burn body fat. Lean muscle is high maintenance when it comes to your metabolism. It's expensive to maintain but that's a good thing. It uses more calories at rest, when you're at your desk, and when you're asleep.

"But Gav, I only want to lose weight, I don't want to be huge and ripped like one of those bodybuilders!"

Relax. I'm not talking about turning you into a huge, muscular bodybuilder. I've been trying hard for the last 20 years to become big, strong, and ripped. It's bloody hard work. If you've got genetics that would make Brad Pitt jealous and you train hard five times per week consistently for the next 10 years, and you eat 3000-5000kcal per day split over five meals, every day; and you take a boat load of PED's (performance enhancing drugs) then you just MIGHT become huge and ripped. Unless that's you, you've got nothing to worry about.

Becoming huge after a bit of weight training is akin to going for a jog this week and setting a world record for the marathon next week. It ain't gonna happen. Small side note here. Eliud Kipchoge's world record time in the marathon of 2hrs.01.39secs is simply amazing isn't? Just to put that into perspective, his average 5km pace was around 14min.24secs but he did eight of those and a bit more in a row. Superhuman. I digress. Back to building muscle. Please, don't fear building muscle. I promise you, the few kgs that you pack onto your frame is your ticket to accelerated fat loss.

We've established that lifting weights or resistance training needs to be the bulk of your training but where do you start?

For some of you who haven't moved for years, exercises that use just your own body weight would be a great place to start. If you've got 30lbs of body fat or more to lose, the weight that you're carrying around day to day is more than enough to get you started. The typical exercises to look at could be body weight squats, lunges, and press-ups. These three exercises will actually use every major muscle group in your body. Don't be fooled by thinking body weight movements are easy. The great thing with using your own body weight is that it can be used for beginner, intermediate, and advanced trainers alike.

Before you perform any routine, make sure you are warmed up. Our aim is to get your heart rate elevated, blood pumping to all your muscles and even a slight sweat on. Here's one I like to use.

1000m on a rowing machine.
25 star jumps
10 press-ups
10 lunges (each leg)
25 star jumps

Here are a few examples of body-weight routines:

Novice

A1 – Bodyweight squats x 20
A2 – Press-ups x 10

A3 – Walking lunges x 10 (each leg)
A4 – Plank shoulder taps x 12 (6 each side)
A5 – Star jumps x 30

A1 - A5 is done back to back with no rest. Complete 1 round and rest for 2mins.

Repeat x 2 for 3 rounds in total.

Although this is a novice routine, an experienced trainee could perform the same circuit but increase the reps, perform more rounds and/or decrease the rest period. A simple circuit can be made extremely tough with just a few changes.

Intermediate

A1 - 10 press-ups
A2 - Star jumps x 60 secs.
A3 - 10 jumping lunges (on each leg)
A4 - Star jumps x 60 secs.
A5 – 10 walkouts to plank

A1 - A5 is done back to back with no rest. Complete 1 round and rest for 45 secs.

Repeat x 4 for 5 rounds in total.

Advanced

A1 – Press-ups x 50
A2 – Reverse crunches x 50
A3 – Mountain climbers x 50
A4 – Star jumps x 50
A5 – Body weight squats x 50

Perform 50 reps of each exercise in any order as quickly as you can without any rest. You don't have to do all 50 reps in a row. You might do 20 press ups, move onto star jumps, then back to do another 15 press ups, and so on. Once you've completed the full circuit of 5 sets of 50 reps, rest for two minutes.

Do three rounds in total, starting with a different move each time. 750 reps in total. Just body weight. Try that one and let me know how you get on!

There really is no limit to what you can do with your own body weight. Can you see that with all these routines, we are using as much muscle mass as possible in every exercise? This is the key to making your bodyweight exercises burn the most calories in the shortest amount of time.

For many more bodyweight exercises and routines, go to **www.theghgmethod/bonus** to download my "12 body weight workouts" cheat sheet.

Now let's look at weight training in the gym.

Many men have had some type of experience in the gym. Most of them in my experience have what I call "just dabbled." They've gone in, lifted a few weights here and there, a bit of bench press and a few bicep curls. Maybe a few squats and deadlifts too, but no real structured program. They've trained the "beach muscles". Chest and biceps, or "chesticles" as it's commonly known in the fitness industry. Why? Because every man wants big pecs and guns, and most men are drawn to that the moment they enter the weights room. It's also a well-known fact amongst male gym users that Monday is "International Chest Day". Just so you know.

Maybe you've trained a bit when you were in your 20s but haven't for a while? Maybe you're reasonably proficient and currently train regularly, or perhaps you're a total beginner? Wherever you are and whatever your experience, you will get the best results if you follow a programme with consistency and use the principle I mentioned at the start of this chapter. Compound exercises.

Here's an example of day 1 of an effective program.

Day 1

A1 – Barbell squat 3 x 8. Rest 120 sec.
A2 – Bench press 3 x 8. Rest 120 sec.
A3 – 1 Arm DB Row 3 x 6-8 (each arm) Rest 60 sec.
A4 - Farmers walk 3 x 30 sec. Rest 120 sec.

This workout is a great start for virtually everyone unless you're very advanced. It's a 3-day per week programme and each session shouldn't take you longer than 45 minutes including a warm-up.

To download the full workout and a few others, go to **www.theghgmethod.com/bonus**

I could spend ages going into things like reps, sets, tempo and training frequency but as I said at the beginning of this book, I want to show you the things that will give you the most "bang for your buck". Advanced techniques have a time and a place but are not usually necessary in the beginning.

What I will explain is "progressive overload". The progressive overload principle states, "for a muscle to grow, strength to be gained, performance to increase, or for any similar improvement to occur, the human body must be forced to adapt to a tension that is above and beyond what it has previously experienced". Basically, what this means is that you must do more than you did last time you were in the gym. Lift more weight or do more reps. You could perform an extra set or decrease the rest period. One of the parameters must change or you will stay the same. This principle applies not only to weight training but to cardio too. In fact, it applies to everything in life. If you want to get better at anything you must do something that you haven't done before. There needs to be some resistance. This is where growth occurs. Physically or mentally, if you don't push to beyond what you are currently capable of, you stay the same.

"If you always put limits on everything you do, physical or anything else, it will spread into your work and into your life. There are no limits. There are only plateaus, and you must not stay there, you must go beyond them."

- Bruce Lee -

Cardio

Cardio is short for cardiorespiratory, which basically means using your heart and lungs. People often debate about the type of cardio to perform. What's the best type of cardio to do, how much, when, and is it better than weight training to burn body fat? Cardio burns body fat for sure, but when it comes to weight training there's no comparison. I like to recommend it to my clients as the icing on the cake. That said; let's look at the different types.

HIIT or "High Intensity Interval Training"

This includes activities such as sprints, Tabata, sled pushing and pulling, farmer's walks and various other short, sharp bursts of activity followed by rest and then repeated. It's effective, it doesn't take too long to perform, but it can be very demanding and stressful on the body so needs to be used sparingly.

Tabata training

Japanese scientist Dr. Izumi Tabata and a team of researchers from the National Institute of Fitness and Sports in Tokyo coined the term "Tabata training" when working with ice skating sprinters. I've highlighted Tabata training, as it is one of my favourite high intensity cardio choices because it's time efficient with each workout lasting only four minutes. It's also been shown to have significant benefits to the cardiovascular system, comparable to that of 30-45 minutes of low intensity aerobic exercise.

Here's an example of how it works.

Press ups x 20 sec. Rest 10 sec.
Body weight squats x 20 sec. Rest 10 sec.

This is repeated another three times for four rounds in total. Four minutes of sheer brutality. You can use any two exercises, but I like to use an upper body and a lower body. This style is extremely demanding, as the heart doesn't know where to pump the blood. Upper then lower and back to upper and so on. It's horrible to be honest, but very effective. If you're feeling particularly masochistic, perform an extra four minutes with the following circuit.

Jumping lunges x 20 sec. Rest 10 sec.
Burpees x 20 sec. Rest 10 sec.

Repeat x 3 for 4 rounds in total. Barf a lung up. Enjoy. You're welcome.

LISS or "Low Intensity Steady State"

There are many examples of LISS. Cycling on a bike or walking/running on a treadmill, swimming, jogging, dancing, and anything else you can think of that involves the movement of your body. The choices are endless. It's usually performed at a lower intensity and over a longer time period. 30 to 40 minutes or more. Pick something you enjoy. Don't ever perform something you don't like. The key is to get moving and get a sweat on. Both high and low intensity cardio have plus points and need to be used according to an individual's goals, circumstances and training schedule.

High intensity is fantastic if the client can push himself or herself this hard and has the nutritional support and lifestyle to recover from it. Many clients come to me in a highly stressed state. Their cortisol is already high. It may not be appropriate to give them high intensity work because this will exacerbate an existing situation. In this instance, low intensity may be more suitable.

Injuries need to be taken into consideration too. High intensity work usually involves more impact, so be aware of your situation and capabilities. Low intensity works for everyone, but some may find it boring. I call it suicide cardio because the thought of walking on a treadmill for 45 minutes makes me want to kill myself. I'm joking of course, but you get the idea. Both will help you burn body fat. Both help you get into a calorie deficit, and both work, but it all depends on your circumstances.

Is it better to do cardio on an empty stomach first thing in the morning or to do it in a fed state? The debate rages on. For many years, many people including myself believed fasted cardio was "the way". The idea was based on the fact that you've gone to bed and you perform your cardio on an empty stomach. By doing this it was suggested that your fat stores could be utilised for energy while you exercise, as opposed to using the food you eat for breakfast. Makes sense, doesn't it?

To be fair, the fitness and bodybuilding community have pushed this idea forever. In fact, many "pros" still do. It turns out that it makes no difference when you do cardio. The fat loss is the same. Without getting too technical, countless studies have shown that more fat is burnt in the fasted state, but the overall net balance at the end of the day is the same, fasted or fed. What's more important is that it gets done. If you like doing cardio on an empty stomach and you like to train before work, then do that. If you can only get to the gym mid-afternoon, don't worry that your lunch will affect your ability to burn body fat. It won't.

That said, whenever I'm trying to get really lean, I like to go in the morning on an empty stomach. It just feels like it's working better. This feeling can make me work harder, go more often and be more diligent with my nutrition. This tends to lead to more fat loss over time but it's not from the cardio itself. It's the other factors.

This is Pretty NEAT

I wasn't going to include this section in the book. In fact, I added it at the very last minute and I will tell you why. My aim was to give you everything I felt was necessary, with no fluff. I didn't think you needed this, but the funny thing is, now I've included it, I'm left thinking, "How on earth could I leave it out?". On the day in question, my fiancée Alex was at a spa with her mum and I was left holding the baby. Daddy day care in full effect. She was at "The Ned" near Bank in central London redeeming her vouchers given as a birthday present from me. Yea, I know. Brownie points were scored. I was on my second walk of the day with our son, Gabriel. I'd not gone to the gym that morning as Alex left early for London, so I decided to get a little exercise done and took a brisk walk with the pushchair into town, around the canal and back via Sainsbury's. The walk back requires considerably more effort than the walk there, as there is a large hill, about 200m long, starting near Sainsbury's that slowly winds all the way to the top near our house. I was breathing heavily, my heart was pounding, and my legs were burning by the time I reached the top. "Who needs the gym", I said to myself. A bit of shopping, a steep hill, and a 12kg baby is all you need. It was during this climb that I decided that this section of the book would make the final cut.

NEAT is an acronym for "non-exercise activity thermogenesis". That is the energy expended for everything we do that is not sleeping, eating, or any activity like the gym, running, or sport. It includes energy expended walking to work, typing, mowing the lawn, playing with the kids, etc. Trivial physical activities all add up and increase your metabolic rate quite substantially. Many people on their weight loss journey beat themselves up when they don't get to the gym as often as they would like. They don't realise that the one-mile walk to work and back every day is worthwhile. That playing football with the kids for two hours at the weekend all helps the cause. If you can't get to the gym, try getting off the tube a stop earlier. Take the stairs instead of the lift at work. Move your body as much as possible doing things you love with the family. This way, exercise isn't a chore, but spontaneous movement becomes highly valued in the quest for an increased metabolism and fat loss.

12. CREATING THE PERFECT DAY

"Carpe diem. Seize the day. Make your life extraordinary"

- Robin Williams, as teacher John Keating, "Dead Poets Society" -

Have you ever had a day when everything just went right? You got up, felt rested, full of energy, got to work, no traffic or delays on public transport. You're productive, efficient, you ate well and even managed to get some exercise in. You got home, played with the kids, had time to relax and talk to your wife. Went to bed happy, content, and satisfied that you'd had such an amazing day. Maybe you've experienced a day like that before and would like to have that experience every day. Maybe you've never experienced it and can only dream of having a day and a schedule like this. The reality is some people do have most of their days like this, and it's not by chance, it's by design.

Some of you might be saying it's impossible to have a perfect day every day, and you know what? You're correct. It is. But by designing an example of a perfect day and using this as a blueprint to copy, you can engineer your day to be the best it can be as often as possible. Four out of seven days is much better than getting up and hoping it all goes your way by chance. It's going to take some work. You'll have to craft how you want your perfect day to look. Here's an example of my "perfect day" to get you started.

My own perfect day starts at 5am in the morning.

5am: Get up, downstairs, 500ml of water with a pinch of organic sea salt.

5.15am: 45mins of personal development, journaling and coffee.

6am: Write daily newsletter and set social media posts for the day.

7am: Wake up my son Gabriel, change his nappy and play with him.

7.30am: Gym. Every day. Weights/cardio/stretch.

9am: Answer emails, interact with clients, book calls etc.

10am: Breakfast.

10.30am: Time with my son.

12pm: Client coaching calls.

2pm: Lunch.

2.30pm: Writing time.

5.30pm: Facebook live group-coaching, emails etc.

6pm: Bath and bedtime story for Gabriel. No work after 6pm.

7pm: Cook dinner, eat, and chill. 1 episode on Netflix.

9pm: In bed and read. No phone/devices after 9pm.

10pm – Lights out. Sexy time if I get lucky. Or it's my birthday.

What I will say is that the perfect day starts the night before, with a great night's sleep. You can't have a perfect day if your sleep is poor. See chapter 14 for more information on optimising your sleep.

Go to **www.theghgmethod.com/bonus** to download the "perfect day" work sheet. Use the sheet to plan your perfect day. You now have a blueprint of how you want your perfect day to look.

Schedule your workouts in your diary like an appointment at the dentist. Most people hate the dentist. You don't want to go but you never miss the appointment because if you do, your teeth fall out and you get charged if you miss it. It's a necessary evil. Here's a good idea. Every time you schedule a workout and you don't go, send £50 to a charity you don't like. Better still. Send £50 to me. I'll graciously accept this cash every time you mess up. Thanks.

Full credit for the "perfect day formula" goes to one of my mentors and coaches, Mr. Craig Ballantyne, who runs "The Perfect Life" workshop all over the world and wrote the book, "The Perfect Day Formula". Personally, since going on his workshop and crafting my perfect day, I've made some subtle but very impactful changes to my life. I've even stopped having just one glass of wine every night, Monday to Friday. I like having the odd glass of red wine, or two as it very often turned out to be, but I didn't need it and it served no purpose. It made me make poor choices at 9.30pm at night. An extra square of chocolate, an extra handful of nuts or an extra cookie, just because I could. My defences are down after just one glass of wine. It was also affecting the quality of my sleep. I've always slept well, but since I've cut the booze, I sleep deeper and feel more rested when the alarm goes off at 5am. I now stop work at 6pm every day, get off my phone at 9pm, and use no more devices after this time. I'm in bed at 9pm and read for one hour before sleeping.

At the time of writing this it's been 12 weeks since I went on Craig's seminar. I've read six books that have sat on my desk for weeks because I carved that time out before bed. Very often I won't make it to 10pm and hit the light switch at 9.45pm, asleep within two minutes max. I set a goal to write and finish this book in 90 days, and did exactly that, all from creating my perfect day. It enabled me to focus on my priorities and goals, to be proactive rather than reactive.

The chances are you won't have your perfect day every day, but wouldn't it be better to have 300 out of 365 productive and perfect days over the course of the year, instead of waking up in the morning and hoping things go your way? By planning out your perfect day in detail, at the beginning, the chance of you having a better week, month, and year are much higher.

13. THE MORNING ROUTINE

"When you arise in the morning, think of what a precious privilege it is to be alive - to breathe, to think, to enjoy, to love"

- Marcus Aurelius -

We've looked at creating the perfect day. Now let's drill down even deeper and look at the morning. If you master your morning, you can master your day. Everyone has a routine in the morning but perhaps you don't realise it because you've never called it a routine. We're all creatures of habit. The question to ask is, are your habits serving you or hindering you? I've realised that if you can start your day and end your day well, the stuff in the middle tends to go pretty damn well. There are a few non-negotiables for me. These are habits that will serve anyone if you put them to good use. I'm not telling you that you MUST do these things in the morning. I'm suggesting that they might help you, as they've personally helped me.

The start of the day begins the night before. You can't expect to have a productive day if you're going to bed late. Sleep is THE most important factor in our life and without adequate rest and recuperation you just can't function or perform optimally. The adage "sleep when you are dead" is not a good mantra, as poor sleep has been linked to a whole host of degenerative conditions and diseases that will lead to an early death. So catch up on that missed sleep (see more in the section on sleep).

Start your day in the best possible way by drinking a large glass or bottle of water.

500ml of cold water with a pinch of organic sea salt is a great start. Most people will sleep 6-8 hours per night. By the time you wake up you're going to be dehydrated. Rehydrating as soon as possible is essential for optimal performance in the day ahead. Give your body what it needs. I've heard it referred to as "an internal bath". Drink this water before you think of having that first cup of coffee. Why the salt? I've found by adding salt to all the water I drink, I reduce my visits to the toilet. There are many formulas designed to tell you how much water you need. Forget them. Just aim for 2-3 litres each day and you won't go far wrong. If you exercise, drink more and let the colour of your pee guide you. Without the salt, I'm pissing like a racehorse every 30 minutes. The water literally goes straight though me. The salt will help you retain water, hydrate you better and is a valuable source of important minerals. I've found that not only do I not need to go to the loo; I don't need to drink as much.

Avoid Checking Your Phone For the First Hour

Many people check their phone the minute they wake. Twitter, Facebook, Instagram, emails, notifications, and then a quick refresh of the Twitter feed, just in case. A deluge of information that somehow fools us into thinking we're connected to the world. We're addicted and this addiction is slowly disconnecting us from humanity. Massive distractions and time-wasting activities, the never-ending dopamine hit of the little red dot that tells us we are enough, continues to govern our lives. Turn your phone off or put it on airplane mode one hour before you go to bed and put it somewhere you won't go the moment you wake up. There is plenty of time to get sucked into the madness. Use the time in the morning to do some of the things I'm about to talk about here.

Personal Development

Personal development has previously been a bit out there. A bit woowoo. A bit wanky. Tell your average Brit that you're into "self-help" and watch their eyes roll; but more and more people are reaping the rewards. One of my mentors, the late Jim Rohn said, "Work harder on yourself than you do on your job". Read a good book or listen to a podcast. Be motivated and inspired by people doing great things in the world. Learn something new. Listen to a great book on Audible. There is no greater thing than to work on yourself. When you improve, everyone's life around you improves. That means your wife and kids and anyone else that you encounter on a regular basis.

Many people say they'd "love to read more but just don't have the time". Commit to 10 pages of a good book every day instead of scrolling on your phone. Use your commute time, which is dead time, to listen and learn. Just 30 minutes per day will make all the difference to your life. Don't know anything about nutrition and losing weight? Read, listen, and learn about it. Teach yourself. One book a month equals 12 books in a year. In five years, you've read 60 books. That's more than 99% of the population will ever read in a lifetime. In five years, you could be virtually an expert in anything you choose. That's the power of personal development. Not so wanky when you break it down, is it? Not sure where to start? One of my favourite books and the most recommended by me to my clients is *"The Slight Edge"* by Jeff Olson. Grab it on Amazon. Whilst you're there, buy another copy of this book and give it to a friend. Thanks.

Hop over to **www.theghgmethod.com/bonus** to download a list of my top 12 recommended books on health, nutrition and mindset.

Write in a Journal

For many, the act of writing in a journal just feels weird. It did for me. What do I write? How much? How do I write? All questions that most people have when they start journaling.

Here are a few things that I write and have helped me:

Plan Your Day

Write your goals & intentions for the day. What are the three biggest things you must achieve to make today a success? Don't call it your "to do" list. Call it your "goals and intentions". Same list but goals and intentions are way more empowering.

Daily Wins & Successes

Write down five "wins" from the day before, however small. Maybe you got to the gym, ate well, and completed a project at work. Great. Write it down. These little successes send a powerful message to your subconscious mind telling you, "You're a winner". The more you do this, the more powerful it becomes. Five wins per day equates to 35 wins for the week. If someone asks you if you had a great week, now you know the answer. Don't underestimate this habit. When you win daily, you want to win even more. Momentum builds and this will spill over into every area of your life.

"The 3 x 3 Formula"

Full credit for this goes to Paul Mort or "Uncle Morty" as he's affectionately known. He specialises in coaching men and he taught me this very handy technique at one of his seminars. Write down three people that you love, three people that love you, and three "things" that you are excited and most proud about. Grab that pen and paper again and fill in the three sections.

Three people that I love are:

_____

Three people that love me are:

_____

Three "things" that I'm excited and most proud about are:

_____

An Attitude of Gratitude

Write down three things you're grateful for. We all have our problems. Some big and some small but if you are reading this you have a lot to be grateful for. Someone somewhere today would love to have your worst day. We often forget how grateful we should be and how lucky we are to have been born where we were. When you're being grateful, you can't be upset or angry. Take a few minutes each day to appreciate this. Go ahead and write below three things you're grateful for:

1:

_____

2:

_____

3:

_____

Whilst you're journaling make sure you do this next point…

Drink a decent cup of coffee

Ahhh Coffee. The elixir of life. Well, maybe not quite, but good organic coffee in the morning is a must (if you like coffee, that is). If you don't, I'm not expecting you to start drinking it now, but I will be honest with you; I don't trust anyone that doesn't drink coffee. I'm joking, but if you do like coffee, you and I will get along fine and dandy. Drink decent quality coffee and don't use instant coffee granules. It tastes like shit and isn't good for you. Personally, I wouldn't go as far to say that coffee is a "health food" but it definitely has some substantial health benefits.

Coffee contains caffeine, as I'm sure you know, which is the most commonly consumed psychoactive substance in the world. Many controlled studies in humans show that coffee improves various aspects of brain function including memory, mood, vigilance, energy levels, reaction times, and general mental function. According to a large review of 18 studies in a total of 457,922 people, each daily cup of coffee was associated with a 7% reduced risk of type 2 diabetes. Coffee is also rich in powerful antioxidants that are believed to be protective against aging and many diseases that are partly caused by oxidative stress, including cancer. Go for organic whenever possible. The conventional coffee bean is one of the most heavily chemically treated crops in the world. It is steeped in synthetic fertilisers, pesticides and herbicides that are potentially harmful to us as humans.

I could spend a lot longer just on this topic, but I won't. Just go organic whenever you can. The bottom line is, coffee is an enjoyable drink for many people with numerous health benefits, so don't shy away from drinking two or three cups per day if you want. As always, the devil is in the dose. Eight double-shot espressos in a day are likely to leave most people staring at the ceiling at 3am.

14. WHO'S THE DADDY?

"I'm trying to give up sexual innuendos, but it's hard. So hard"

- Someone -

This is one of the most important chapters in this book. The body is governed by several hormones, which can either help or hinder you on your weight loss journey. Having a reasonable level of understanding of these hormones will be very beneficial for you. Let's start with the king himself…

Testosterone

Testosterone is the primary male sex hormone that plays many important roles in the body. In men, it regulates libido (sex drive), bone mass, fat distribution, muscle mass, strength, production of red blood cells, and production of sperm. It's the daddy of all hormones when it comes to losing fat and building muscle. Anyone you know who is in great shape has a high testosterone level naturally or is taking an exogenous supply of testosterone in the form of anabolic steroids or some other performance enhancing drugs. Women have testosterone too, but the average male will have 15 times more than the average woman, which is why men are generally stronger than women, with more muscle mass and less body fat.

With high T levels bringing more muscle, less body fat, increased aggression and an increased sex drive, you can see why the pursuit of higher levels is so important to many men, especially professional athletes and sportsmen. Low levels of testosterone have been linked to low energy and depression, lack of motivation, increased chances of obesity, and an increased risk of disease and premature death. That's not even mentioning the fatty deposits, lack of strength, and decreased ability to achieve and maintain an erection.

I don't know about you but having a penis that only reaches "half-mast" or only works sporadically is not my idea of fun. If losing more fat, building more muscle, increasing motivation, confidence, and all-around performance in life, *AND* having lead in your pencil sounds like your cup of tea, this is the section of the book for you.

How Do We Increase Testosterone?

No 1: Exercise and lifting weights

Exercise is one of the most effective ways to prevent many lifestyle related diseases, but it can also boost your testosterone. Resistance training and lifting heavy weights is the best type of exercise to boost T levels. Studies show that a heavy set of high rep squats (15-20) can raise your testosterone significantly. Focus on compound movements: movements that utilize as much muscle mass as possible. This boosts testosterone, builds muscle, and burns fat. Increased testosterone means less body fat and more muscle, which leads to an increase in the weights you can lift. This continues to go full circle with each mechanism feeding the other. It's a win-win.

No 2: Diet and nutrition

Your diet has a major influence on testosterone, as well as other important hormones but for now we will focus on testosterone. Adequate protein can help to maintain and increase muscle mass, which will in turn increase your levels of testosterone. A diet rich in healthy fats such as avocado, olive oil, nuts, seeds, cold-water fish like salmon as well as saturated fats from sources such as beef and coconut oil have been shown to boost T-levels. Contrary to popular belief, a diet rich in fat is one of the best things you can do to improve your health.

No 3: Minimise stress and cortisol levels

Cortisol is an important hormone when it comes to testosterone. When cortisol is raised, T levels are lowered.

Go to **www.theghgmethod.com/bonus** to download the "Stress Free" Cheat Sheet and discover the best ways to reduce stress.

No 4: Vitamin D levels and sun exposure

Vitamin D is a crucial nutrient in boosting and optimising your overall health as well as testosterone. Vitamin D can be obtained from your diet. Tuna, mackerel, salmon, cheese, egg yolks, and beef liver all contain good amounts of vitamin D, although it's very difficult to achieve optimal levels from food alone. Supplementation is usually required, and of course adequate sunlight exposure is also needed. Despite its importance, nearly half the population of the US is deficient in vitamin D, and if you live in northern Europe, you can forget about it. There just isn't enough sunlight to expose yourself to. It's highly likely your vitamin D level will be deficient. A recent study showed that supplementing with around 3000 IUs of vitamin D per day increased T-levels by 25%.

No 5: Other vitamin and mineral supplements

In one study, zinc and vitamin B supplements increased sperm quality by 74% and zinc has been shown to increase T levels at least in those deficient in zinc. Other studies suggest vitamins A, C, and E can play a role, but more research is needed.

No 6: BPAs

Limit exposure to oestrogenic chemicals found in cleaning and personal care products, tap water, and BPAs. BPA (Bisphenol A) is a chemical that is added to many commercial products including food containers and hygiene products.

No 7: Sleep

Sleep is so important. In relation to maximising testosterone, there can be no debate. The University of Chicago took a group of lean healthy young males in their mid-twenties and limited them to 5 hours of sleep per night for one week. They tested the blood of the participants and the results were astonishing. The results showed that the marked drop effectively "ages a man by 10-15 years in terms of testosterone virility".

Men who report sleeping too little or having poor sleep quality have a 29% lower sperm count than those getting a decent night's kip. More importantly perhaps, they also have significantly smaller testicles than those who sleep well. If maximising your efforts at the gym, burning fat, and the size of your balls holds your attention in even just a remote way, getting quality sleep should be high on your agenda.

No 8: Reduce alcohol intake

I'm not saying give up alcohol entirely, but I'm saying reduce intake if testosterone production is important to you. The devil, as always, is in the dose. I get it, you like a drink. You work hard and your life is stressful. You don't sleep much because of work and family commitments. I'm not saying that this is going to be easy, far from it. But if you want to achieve some level of efficiency in the gym and your life, then getting a grip on lifestyle factors that affect your testosterone is paramount.

I had a client called Chris. He really struggled to lower his body fat and get lean. He was in reasonable shape (his words), but just couldn't seem to lose those love handles. He'd seen a hint of his abs once, but a six-pack was a long way away. His diet was okay, he trained three times per week, but he boozed quite heavily, drinking about 20 to 30 units per week. I suggested that we get his testosterone tested. It's quite a simple test available on Amazon. A quick saliva sample was sent off and the results were back in a week or so. The result was a real eye opener for Chris. The test alone caused him to decrease his boozing. He focused on his nutrition and sleep. We re-tested his testosterone 12 weeks later. Not only were his T levels way above normal for a man of his age (38), he lost 18 pounds of body fat, and his performance in the gym increased dramatically. That's the power of increased testosterone.

Chris' Testimonial:

"I just couldn't seem to get the results I wanted, and I knew it was probably down to my drinking. I reluctantly took the testosterone test that Gav suggested and was shocked by the results. Because of this, I cut my drinking by at least half and noticeably saw the difference in my body in a few weeks. I felt stronger, had more energy and lost body fat. Without going into too much detail, the Mrs said that she noticed a difference in the bedroom too. I'll take that. Thanks Gav".

15. SLEEP, ALCOHOL, STRESS, & IMPORTANT HORMONES

"Sleep is the best meditation"

- Dalai Lama -

Sleep

We all know sleep is important, but do we realize how, why, and to what extent? Many of you reading this may think sleep is just a time machine to bring you to breakfast tomorrow. In a way you'd be right, but that's not the whole story. I've shown you how important sleep is for the production of testosterone, but there's much more. Sleep plays an important role when losing weight and getting in shape, but more importantly perhaps, it is crucial for your mental, physical, and emotional health and wellbeing.

Sleeping less than six or seven hours a night can suppress your immune system and more than doubles your risk of cancer. In fact, shift workers have higher rates of obesity, diabetes, and cancer, and the World Health Organization has classified shift work as a probable carcinogen, which means there's a potential to cause cancer. Insufficient sleep is a key factor in determining whether you may develop Alzheimer's and can increase the risk of cardiovascular disease, stroke, and heart failure. Many people just don't sleep well, that's a fact, but it doesn't have to be that way.

I'll show you how to improve your sleep dramatically but first let's look at some of the things in life that can disrupt your sleep. Poor diet, and alcohol consumption play big roles. Stress from work and family life cause people to lose sleep. The use of smartphones and other devices that emit blue light, which interfere with your circadian rhythm and the production of melatonin (the 'sleep hormone'), all contribute to the quality of your night's sleep. Just one night of bad sleep can radically increase cortisol levels and suppress melatonin. This cortisol can break down your muscle tissue by converting muscle into glucose through a process called gluconeogenesis and put your body into "fight or flight" mode. Not only will this affect your ability to sleep well, it also affects your ability to build or maintain muscle mass.

Let's look at sleep in relation to losing weight and your metabolism.

Lack of sleep plays havoc with two other key hormones; leptin and ghrelin. Aside from sounding like two characters from "The Lord of the Rings", they're responsible for controlling your appetite and weight. Leptin sometimes called the "satiety hormone" is produced in your fat cells. It's basically responsible for the feeling of being full. When Leptin is high, you feel satisfied. When it's low, you want to eat more. Its not so distant cousin ghrelin is known as the "hunger hormone". It stimulates your appetite and increases hunger and food intake, which can in turn promote fat storage and weight gain.

Many studies have shown that inadequate sleep decreases concentrations of this satiety signaling hormone leptin, while increasing levels of ghrelin, the appetite and hunger instigator. Not only is the desire to eat much more prevalent when you haven't slept enough, your body is saying it's not full. It's like being totally out of control of your own desire to eat and knowing when to stop. If you've ever been trapped in this vicious cycle, it's not fun at all. If weight loss is important to you, you must gain control of these important hormones.

Go to **www.theghgmethod.com/bonus** to download my "Sleep Cheat Sheet" to massively improve the quality of your sleep.

My client Phil was a terrible sleeper. Busy and stressed at work, six coffees most days and a lot of junk food. He also liked two or three beers most nights to unwind at home. Two or three probably meant three or four and maybe more. It was no surprise to me that the quality of his sleep was terrible. Going to bed late (midnight), up twice in the night to take a pee and finding it hard to get back to sleep, he'd wake up feeling exhausted. Using my "sleep cheat sheet" he radically changed the quality of his sleep.

Phil's testimonial:

"Gav told me to reduce my coffee intake from six cups to just two cups and never after 4pm. This was hard for me as I realise now I was using this coffee to keep me awake. I stopped drinking Monday to Thursday, and I started turning my phone and laptop off completely at 8pm. To be honest, the changes in my sleep quality were dramatic, almost immediately. These changes might seem easy for many, but they were very hard for me in the beginning. I was determined to follow it through, and I have Gav to thank for helping me with this".

Alcohol

Most people like and enjoy the odd glass of alcohol now and then, but few of us would argue that it's the most conducive habit when it comes to health and fitness. That said, you could drink alcohol and still lose body fat, but more on that in a minute. Previously I mentioned how too much alcohol can lower testosterone levels. When testosterone is reduced, it's harder to burn fat and build muscle. Less muscle can mean a lower metabolic rate, which could in turn lead to an increase in fat storage, the exact opposite of what we're trying to achieve. There are 7kcal per gram of alcohol compared to 4kcal per gram of protein and carbs, and 9kcal per gram of fat. The problem isn't necessarily with this number. It's the fact that they are empty calories that contain no nutrients to aid the body in any way, and once consumed, they effectively put the body on pause. Alcohol calories cannot be stored for later so they must be used immediately.

Your metabolic system literally stops and processes the alcohol before resuming its normal functions. It's very easy to add hundreds if not thousands of calories to your body through alcohol. On top of that, alcohol lowers the inhibitions, lowers your blood sugar, and can increase your appetite.

Your resolve to avoid the canapés and other calorie-laden snacks at a dinner party mixed with a cavalier attitude of "fuck it", and an increase in appetite can often create a disastrous situation. "Just one" has probably been the downfall of everyone at some point in his or her life. Just one invariably leads to another, and another. Not only are you getting excess calories from the alcohol, you're adding more into the mix from the very tasty but largely useless, high calorie, fat-laden processed snacks. You haven't even started on the buffet yet. Calories aside, too much alcohol is just bad for your health. Alcohol can affect the quality of your sleep. Drinking may fool you into thinking you're sleeping well, but you're sedated rather than falling into a deep sleep. After drinking you spend more time in REM sleep, which is rapid eye movement. This can leave you feeling tired no matter how long you stay in bed.

Alcohol irritates your digestive system. Even just a glass or two can cause your stomach to produce more acid than usual, leading to inflammation of the stomach lining. Every drink serves an increased risk of cancer of the mouth, tongue, lip, throat, stomach, pancreas, and colon. Drinking also makes it more difficult to digest food and absorb vital nutrients, particularly protein and vitamins.

Alcohol, as I mentioned before, lowers your inhibitions and seriously affects your decision-making capabilities. Your sudden drive to sleep with the closest female near you, regardless of how attractive she is could cause a problem if you have a girlfriend or wife. Many men have fallen victim to the incredibly common phenomenon known as "beer goggles". I'm not making excuses for it, or condoning it, I'm making you aware that it's a thing. Pay attention. Alcohol can make you fat, screw with your health and fuck up your marriage. Don't say I didn't warn you.

Enough of the doom and gloom. If you're a heavy drinker, my advice is to reduce it. Firstly, from a health perspective and secondly if burning body fat and losing weight is a concern. You just don't need those excess empty calories, do you? I think we all know the answer to that.

Here's my top tip to reduce your intake. Choose alcohol-free days. Pick three or four days per week where you don't have a drink. Take note of how you feel. You should feel improvements, but it will take time to really see the benefits. If you have a few events during the week have a strict cut off point with the time and amount you drink. For example, you could say I'm going to have three drinks and the last one will be by 9pm. This will minimise the damage and help with your sleep.

Stress - The Silent Killer

I'd like you take this next section very seriously. Stress has been called the "silent killer" for a reason. I thought I would show you how to recognize it and give you some effective strategies to cope with it. You know what stress is, don't you? Stress on the body can come from many sources, such as synthetic substances like alcohol, drugs, and tobacco, pollution - especially if you live in the city, and just the general pace of work, family, and life. One area of stress we don't always think of, or even recognize, is the food we eat. Even so-called "healthy food" can be laden with antibiotics and pesticides that put your body under significant stress over time.

A very brief science lesson: When we're stressed our bodies produce and release the chemicals adrenalin and cortisol, amongst others, which basically puts our body into "fight or flight" mode. For our Neanderthal ancestors, hundreds of thousands of years ago, this mode was essential for survival and would have saved many from sabre-tooth tiger attacks or nocturnal invasions to the cave from other tribes. This stress was not a problem (assuming they were still alive) as once the attack or stress had subsided, the hormones released would dissipate and normal life would continue.

In the modern era, stress accumulates from non-life-threatening problems and can continue to mount up. Unless effective stress reducing activity is implemented, it can cause you serious short and long-term problems. Short-term problems can include poor sleep, low mood, depression, low sex drive, poor digestion, bowel suppression, fluid retention, and weight gain. There are a lot more, but I tried to keep it relevant. Long-term problems could include a high risk of degenerative diseases such as arthritis, diabetes, cancer, stroke, and heart disease. Not fun at all. So, what can we do to minimise stress and effectively combat it, so life happens for you and not to you?

Recent studies have shown that the perceived level of stress was more dangerous than the actual stress itself. If someone is consistently telling him or herself, "I'm stressed", this can be more damaging than someone with the same level of stress who is mentally able to cope better. It's probably wise to reduce the burden of stress rather than focusing too much on the mental side of things. So, what can we do to reduce stress? There are many ideas and techniques, but I've boiled them down to 10 that I've personally used on myself and recommend to clients with great success.

Go to **www.theghgmethod/bonus** to download a FREE cheat sheet on the top 10 things you can do right now to reduce your stress levels.

I hope those of you that are feeling stressed can implement these ideas into your daily routine. Now, excuse me. I need to go sit in the lotus position in an Epsom salt bath and meditate whilst drinking a protein shake and an intravenous supply of super greens and fish oil. OMMMMMM. Namaste. (If you have no idea what I'm talking about then you need to go and download the cheat sheet)

Hormones

I want to touch on hormones a little more. I don't want you to get too bogged down with this, but it's important to have a basic understanding of hormones; what they are and how they work in the body, so you can control them, rather than them controlling you. There are about 50 different hormones, which are the chemical messengers of your body created in the endocrine system. These messengers control most major bodily functions from basic needs like hunger, to complete systems like reproduction, emotions, and biological needs. I want to look at three key ones: insulin, leptin, and ghrelin. We had a cursory look at leptin and ghrelin a little earlier so let's start with insulin.

Insulin is produced in the pancreas and regulates the amount of glucose in the blood. It allows your body to use sugar (glucose) from the food you eat for energy, or to store that energy for future use. It also helps to keep your blood sugar from getting too high (hyperglycemic), or too low (hypoglycemic).

Have you ever eaten something high in sugar and felt great but in an hour or so you felt starving, irritable, sluggish, and even quite weak? This is the classic insulin spike and drop. Let's say you eat cornflakes and drink a glass of orange juice for breakfast. If you grew up in the 70s or 80s you definitely had that type of breakfast at least once in your life. To be honest, many people are still eating this now. You can substitute cornflakes for any high carb sugary cereal; they're all the same. You eat your breakfast at 7am. Your blood sugar gets ramped up. Your pancreas releases insulin to deal with the sugar and bring it back down, often overshooting and taking it too low. You've crashed. What do you do? You reach for more sugar to bring you back up and this rollercoaster of hunger, irritability, and uncontrollable emotions continues.

Very often I hear clients tell me, "I just can't stop eating carbs. I need them". On closer analysis of their diet it turns out to be that they've got on this rollercoaster early in the day and can't get off. For years, many health and fitness professionals, including myself, thought insulin was the culprit for people gaining weight. It's a fat storage hormone, but it's also highly anabolic, meaning it both builds muscle and helps to store fat.

Allow me to explain…

Hormones will drive your behaviour, but ultimately, calorie intake will trump hormones any day of the week. A massive influx of simple sugars will spike your insulin levels; there is no question of that. If someone is in a calorie deficit for the day or the week, that insulin spike won't make him or her store body fat. That high carb meal will release hormones (insulin) that may cause you to make a poor choice for your next meal, which could result in an overconsumption of calories for the day, but it may not.

Here is an extreme example. Let's say someone ate four bowls of corn flakes with milk, spaced evenly over the day with a total of 800kcal for the day. Cornflakes and milk are like little insulin time bombs going off in your body. Blood sugar goes sky high, insulin does its job, but with only 800kcal intake for the day, would that person gain weight? The answer is no. They can't without a calorie surplus.

Too many calories will cause someone to gain weight, regardless of insulin or not. There is a fair chance that person may be irritable, hungry, tired, and not satisfied. But if they stopped at 800 calories a day on the cornflake diet, they'd lose a tonne of weight. Disclaimer: I'm not telling anyone to actually do this. This is purely to give you an extreme scenario. My sincerest apologies to all the bowls of cornflakes around the world. I picked on you. I'm sorry. It's not personal. I like you. You just served as a great example.

So, that's insulin. Be aware of what it's doing in your body. Making better food choices will help you to avoid that rollercoaster in the first place. As I mentioned the cornflake breakfast and what *not* to do, I thought I should give you some examples of what you could do.

I had a client called Jack that was stuck on that rollercoaster and really struggled to get off. He was eating a very high carb, nutrient deficient breakfast every morning. Monday to Friday he would drink a large glass of orange juice before he left the house at around 6.30am and on arrival into the city at 8am, he would grab a croissant filled with chocolate and a large milky cappuccino with three sugars and a sprinkle of chocolate on top. It's safe to say he had conditioned his body into expecting sugar. He couldn't work out why he was always starving before lunch, or why his concentration levels and productivity were not where they should be. In short, he was feeling hungry all the time. I suggested we change his breakfast; he was open to my suggestions. I told him to aim for protein and a good source of fat in the morning. This would regulate his blood sugar and give him a nice steady flow of energy, without the ups and downs, all the way to lunchtime. "Three scrambled eggs and some smoked salmon or avocado could be a good choice. Maybe some berries added into the mix".
Starting the day with a breakfast that is protein rich and contains a good amount of essential fats will produce a vastly different output in results for

most people in terms of energy, satiety, and mental acuity. This enables a person to make wiser choices for the rest of the day, which in terms of fat loss, is the key. You take control of the choices you make and don't allow your hormones to drive you.

The Secret Weapons: Leptin and Ghrelin

These guys are both important players in regulating appetite. I mentioned in chapter 16 how poor sleep can play havoc with this system, but let's look at these two hormones a little closer. If you have a small understanding of how these two work, your chance of losing weight and staying in shape will be considerably higher. It's fair to say that many people that go on a diet and lose weight end up regaining that weight over the next few months or years. The body doesn't like change. It will always try to maintain some sort of homeostasis. When dieting, calorie consumption goes down and our body responds by making us hungrier. It's quite clever when you think about it. From a purely survival point of view, our bodies do exactly what they're designed to do. Hormones kick in and make us want to eat more.

Leptin decreases hunger. Ghrelin increases hunger. Here lies the problem. Both hormones get messed up with obesity. Leptin is produced by adipose tissue (body fat). Leptin tells the brain we have enough fat, are satisfied, so we can eat less or skip eating. The more fat you have, the more leptin you make, so you would think that people with more fat to lose would magically stop eating and lose weight. But this is where it gets a little unfair. The brain doesn't hear this signal. It downregulates its receptors and essentials 'stops listening' to the hormone telling your body to decrease appetite. There's no increase in metabolism, and your body may think that no leptin is being produced. This is called leptin-resistance. It makes you hungrier. A horrible, vicious cycle. It's not your fault. Being overweight or having excess body fat can mess up your appetite signals and make you hungrier.

Ghrelin is produced in the stomach when it's empty. It screams at you to eat more food. It's high before you eat, and low after you eat. You can see that if you want to lose weight, you want less ghrelin, so you don't get hungry. Both hormones regulate appetite and hunger and will self-regulate with the aim of keeping you in the same place you are now. When you try to lose body fat, your hormone levels change and make you hungry again. This situation can lead to the dreaded yo-yo effect, which is very common when dieting.

So that's a brief look at a few important hormones. But what can you do with this info? Well, you will hopefully be able to recognise how you feel and realise that you dictate how these hormones work and use them to your advantage, rather than letting them control you. Eating a super high carbohydrate breakfast may make you ravenously hungry a few hours later. Now you know why, and if that's you, you can make a better choice first thing in the morning. Getting a poor night's sleep will mess with your leptin and ghrelin. Now you know this. Before you just knew you were hungry and craved carbohydrates. Armed with this knowledge you can work on your sleep patterns or at least understand that you will seek those high carb options like a bloodhound on the scent for wild boar. YOU are in control. You can control your hormones with the choices you make with your lifestyle. Once you master this, life becomes fun. You're no longer on that emotional rollercoaster of hunger, diets, and deprivation. It's a nice place to be. Once you get there, you will realise just how easy this can be.

16. SELF-LIMITING BELIEFS & YOUR MINDSET

"Whether you think you can or think you can't, you're right"

- Henry Ford -

The dictionary definition of a belief is something you can trust, have faith and confidence in. You see what you believe; you don't believe what you see. We see the world through our own filter. This filter has been constructed from our past experiences, good and bad. This means that many of the things we believe in or believe to be true may not actually be so. If you believe something and you experience it, you'll always find evidence or ideas to support that belief, even if it's not true. It could be a story. A story we've told ourselves repeatedly. This story could be positive and empowering but very often it's negative and disempowering. It can often be destructive, demotivating, and demoralising.

In the context of health, fitness, and weight loss, I often hear extremely negative self-limiting beliefs. Here are some classic examples. "I can't lose weight". "I've got big bones". "I've tried everything". "It's hereditary". "I've got a slow metabolism". "I'm no good". "I don't deserve it". "I have never been slim" and many, many more. The truth is very often entirely different. In nearly all the clients I've worked with over the last 20 years, these beliefs were made up in their own heads and told with such frequency that they became real.

"I've tried everything".

Well, you haven't tried everything because if you had, you would have lost weight. The truth is you've tried a few things and they didn't work. Maybe you've tried many things and you quit before they worked, or maybe they were just stupid ideas in the first place. These failures have given you enough evidence to convince you this is true.

"I told you so" becomes the attitude. The self-limiting belief quickly becomes a self-fulfilling prophecy. You get exactly what you expect. This vicious cycle continues with no hope of you breaking out of the cycle. Your experiences, beliefs, and life have literally programmed you.

How do we change these beliefs? You need a new programme. Jim Rohn said, "We are the average of the five people we spend the most time with". Your environment and the people in that environment shape and mould you. You become like these people. Your parents and your childhood. Your schooling and your peers. Every person you've ever met and every single interaction, good or bad, has brought you to where you are today, right now.

If you're trying to lose weight and your family and friends like to eat and drink a lot, you'll find it quite hard to shake that influence. On the flip side, if you spend time with people that support your goals; who eat healthily, your chances increase significantly in achieving those goals. You might be thinking, "Oh, I need to ditch all my fat friends". No, I'm not saying that. I am saying limit your exposure to them and increase the time you spend with people that are fit and healthy. This can make a huge difference. Read books on health and fitness. Influences and mentors are not limited to people you know in person. There is an inexhaustible supply of books available to you in bookshops and online. Use these resources. Soak up the vast amount of information that someone else took years and maybe a lifetime to experience and put down on paper. It's all there for you. Educate yourself. Be inspired by greatness.

Avoid Reading the Newspapers and Watching the News

Someone says, "I need to know what's going on in the world!" Do you? Do you really? You need to know that a typhoon just wiped out 2,000 people in the Philippines? You need to know an aircraft just crashed into the sea killing all 360 passengers and crew, many of whom were children. The truth is we DON'T need to know this, but we like it. It's addictive. Newspapers are not designed to inform you. They're designed to shock you and report the latest scandal or tragedy and as humans we lap it up. We can't get enough of it. I counted the ratio of negative to positive stories in the first 20 pages of a well-known newspaper here in the UK. There was a 10:1 ratio in favour of doom and gloom. The truth is, all around us there are millions of great things that happen all the time, but it doesn't grab your attention. It doesn't pull you in and shock you.

A Monk & A Ferrari

Six years ago, I picked up a book from my bookcase called 'The Monk Who Sold His Ferrari' by Robin Sharma. I'd previously read the book in 1997, but like many books back in my early 20s, I discarded it and took nothing from it. Fast-forward to 2012, I reread the book and it was like the lights went on. You will have heard the phrase, "when the student is ready, the teacher will appear". Well, this student was more than ready to soak up everything he could get his hands on. I looked a little further into Robin Sharma on YouTube and found two videos that stood out to me. One was called 'The 5am Club' and the second one was 'How To Journal'. These were separate videos but the two are inextricably linked.

Robin said, "All great performers, thought leaders, successful business owners, and entrepreneurs get up at 5am and work on themselves".

Now, whether the 5am alarm clock is entirely true or not, is irrelevant. To be fair, it probably isn't but what he was saying was that most successful people in all walks of life, get up early, plan the day and work on their own personal development by reading, watching, or listening to ideas and strategies to improve their life. Positive, uplifting, inspirational, and motivational words. Wisdom and thoughts from some of the great leaders of our civilisation. Past and present. Alive and dead.

That's what I did for three straight months, missing only a few days. I got up at 5am every morning. I aimed to be in bed at 10pm. If I was late, I was still up at 5am. If it was midnight, I was up at 5am. On the weekends, I was up at 5am and would spend the three hours from 5am to 8am, reading, learning, listening, and improving myself. It wrecked my social life, but I was on a mission.

On only five hours sleep some days, I was extremely tired, but I just got up, despite my tiredness. I wore the lack of sleep like a badge of honour. Admittedly, there were times when I should have slept more but I was totally immersed in self-improvement and bettering myself like I never had before. I've never worked as hard and enjoyed the process as I did in these three months. I wrote in my journal all the things I was learning. I learnt how to write goals and why they're so important. I learnt how to be grateful for the things I currently had, while still striving to improve other areas of my life.

It was during this time I learnt to not read the newspapers. For a whole year, I never looked at a newspaper for more than a quick glance. I will be honest. I missed it. I loved reading the newspaper and still do, but I avoided it and guess what? I still knew what was happening in the world. I was still informed enough but by limiting my exposure to all the negativity, my outlook in life changed tremendously. This has been a very long-winded way of saying that the only reason you're reading this book is because I worked on myself. I was exposed to greatness daily. I listened and learned. Amazing people inspired me. I believed writing a book was possible. I saw evidence of people with far less than I have achieving incredible things. People with less education, money, and resources achieving unbelievable success, and I thought if they can, why not me?

I chose not to believe the stories in my head. Stories like "who am I to think I can write a book? Why would anyone read my book? Only famous people write good books. Am I good enough? Can I even write a book?"

All self-limiting beliefs and bullshit stories. Working on my own personal development enabled me to realize that you can pretty much do anything you set as a goal, if you work towards it every day and believe you can do it. I'm trying to suggest that by exposing yourself to the right information, ideas, and surrounding yourself with the right people, you CAN change your current negative beliefs into beliefs that will enable you to achieve incredible results in any area of your life, including weight loss.

Look at some of your own self-limiting beliefs regarding weight loss right now. We all have them. I know you have them too. Below write down three self-limiting beliefs about why you can't lose weight. This can be tough if you've never consciously thought about these, never mind written them down.

Here are a couple of mine to get you started.

1. I can't write a book. I don't have the skills or the knowledge to write a book.

2. People will think I'm stupid, have a disability and think that I'm not attractive when they know I wear hearing aids.

Both complete rubbish. That I do know. In fact, I always knew it deep down, but it didn't stop me playing the story over and over in my head for years. OK, now it's your turn. Don't be shy. The first step to mastery is admitting weakness. There is strength in vulnerability.

Go ahead and write down 3 self-limiting beliefs about your weight loss and health.

1:

_____

2:

_____

3:

_____

Stop Making Excuses.

I've tried everything. I just can't lose weight. I've got big bones; we all have in my family. There is a history of depression in our family. I've got a slow metabolism. I have an under-active thyroid gland. I don't like exercise. I bulk up too quickly. Whenever I do weight training, I put on too much muscle. I just want to tone up. I don't want to get too big. I need carbohydrates. It's the weekend and I've been good all week. Red wine is good for the heart. I need motivation. I just can't stop myself. It's not my fault. It's my parents'/spouse's/boss' fault.

It's Not My Fault!

That's probably the biggest excuse known to man. It's also the most disempowering. You must take responsibility for everything in your life whether it's good or bad. You created it. You created it all. In one way or another, where you are in your life financially, emotionally, physically, mentally or in any other way you can possibly think of, it's all down to you and the decisions you made.

I'm not saying you had it easy. Your life may have been tough. It may have been extremely violent or filled with abuse. I'm not judging you or anyone by trying to suggest that it's easy. However, you do have a choice in how to react to these conditions. You have a choice to overcome those problems and difficulties, however wrong, disgusting, and diabolical they are/were. Or you can let them overcome you and rule your life.

Before you shout and scream at this page saying, "what the fuck do you know about a shitty life", I will tell you right now. I know nothing about it. My childhood was great. I had a great family, good education in a great home environment with brilliant parents that loved and supported me throughout my formative and teenage years. I have nothing to complain about. If you compare my life to some people's lives, you would know for sure that life isn't fair. Yet, however awful your existence was, you have a choice in how you react to this right now. How do I know that to be true? Because the evidence is clear to me and to everyone that wants to find it. I can name countless successful people that had every reason to lose the plot. They had every reason to drop out of society and become an addict. Sex, booze or drugs, you choose your poison.

It all comes down to a decision that the individual makes. A decision that says I'm not going to allow external circumstances to determine my success. I'm not going to allow my upbringing and environment to shape how I live the rest of my life. These people decided that despite the odds stacked against them, they wouldn't allow these circumstances to affect how they moved forward in their life. You can decide how to live your life, despite the things that took place before. You can decide if you want to be successful and you can decide if you're going to allow all that shit to shape your future. It's your choice. I know that's hard to hear for some people. Some people have been blaming others their whole lives for why they can't get it together.

"Everybody is self-made, but only the successful will admit it". I love that quote and how true it is. We're all self-made. We created what we have and where we are. You don't like what you have and where you are? Then change it. I can tell you right now, no one else is going to change it for you. No one is coming to the rescue. No one is going to bail you out and make it all OK. Everyone else is far too busy focusing on his or her own shit. No one cares enough to make sure you're OK. Of course, people care about you. I don't mean that no one cares about you in the normal sense, as long as you're safe and have enough to get by. People will help but when it comes down to it, as long as they and theirs are all good, that is their main concern. Not you. So, get over that fact. Stop telling yourself and everybody else that you can't make anything from your life because of the bullshit story you keep telling yourself. The story going on in your head that stops you from taking action. The bullshit story that is on repeat, day after day, night after night, that keeps telling you that you're not good enough.

You are good enough, despite the shit that's happened to you. This stuff does not define you. It doesn't have to create your reality moving forward. It happened. Now choose to move past that and get on with your life. Most people are constantly thinking about the past or worrying about the future. How about living in the present and focusing on the next 24 hours ahead of you? Stop thinking about what someone said or did to you, what someone didn't say to you or how you were let down. Stop it. Look at your day ahead. How can you make this next 24 hours really count? How can you turn what you have into what you want?

Rather than looking at what you don't have in your life, look at what you do have. Look at the skills you possess rather than the skills you don't possess. What skills do you possess? Look at what you have and where you are. Don't blame anyone or anything for what you don't have. That's the blame game. No one wins, and no one cares. Focus on where you want to go and make the best of what you have. If you have laser focus on where you're heading; all the right people, money, and opportunities will show up when you need them. It's just the way it is. The law of attraction is very real. Most people don't understand this and consequently don't make a start. They use every excuse under the sun about why it won't work for them.

I think many people spend too much time working on improving the things they can't do when they should spend their time improving what they're already good at. Focus on your strengths. Don't focus on your weaknesses. There are far too many people in the world that are great at what you suck at. Find those people to work on your weaknesses and spend your time doing the things you're great at. The things that come naturally to you. You know what you're great at, the things that come very easily.

What makes some succeed despite extreme adversity compared to others that lose their grip on life and succumb to the depths of despair? David Goggins is an ex Navy SEAL that overcame tremendous odds to achieve many great things. Here is a young boy that grew up in an abusive family. His father beat his mother and when he saw this happening, his dad beat him too. He was 7 years old when this first happened, and it went on for years. He lived in Indiana in a town that was a KKK stronghold with only a few other African-American families living there. He was called "nigger" every day at school with no protection from the teachers. He was abused physically and mentally every day for most of his childhood. His weight ballooned up to 297lbs at his heaviest. He was morbidly obese, emotionally damaged, working in a job he hated (killing rodents and cockroaches) and thought, "this is it, this is my life".

He had every reason to do nothing and accept his fate. Most wouldn't blame him if he did. But Goggins decided that his life wasn't going to be one of mediocrity. He decided that he wanted more from his life. No one cared. No one helped him, and he realized that nobody was ever coming to the rescue. He was told that he needed to lose 100lbs in three months to become a Navy SEAL. He couldn't run a single mile without gasping for breath. He went on to lose over 100lbs in three months. A few years later, he decided to enter a race. This wasn't your average 5km park run on a Sunday morning. He decided he was going to run 100 miles in less than 24 hours. Ultra-marathons are a thing, and many compete in events like this every week all over the world. But for a guy who didn't do any training, Goggins ran 100 miles in about 19 hours. Later he went on to compete in many other ultra-marathons and extreme endurance events, including breaking the world record for completing 4,030 pull-ups in 17 hours. He did all of this despite shitty childhood circumstances and the fact that he used to weigh 297lbs. David Goggins should have been a statistic. He decided otherwise.

I could spend the next 20 pages of this book telling you about people that overcame extreme circumstances and have achieved greatness, but I won't. There is no need. Wherever you are in your life, whatever has happened to you, you must realise that this doesn't need to define you. You can still be successful and achieve what you want with your health, fitness, fat loss, and anything else in life that you put your mind to. You have the power to do this. You have the power right now to change your life in any way you want. All it takes is a decision. A snap of the fingers. A heartbeat. The choice is yours.

Don't Compare Yourself To Others

With the world of social media dominating many people's lives today it's sometimes hard to not compare yourself to others. What you must realise is that the "one shot selfie" was taken 36 times and the "no make-up selfie" is still made up slightly. The "woke up looking like this selfie" is also a fake; just like the Breitling you bought in that Turkish souk last year on holiday.

We all want to look and feel good in life, I know that, but much of what we see these days just isn't the truth. Even if it was true, comparing yourself to others is futile and will serve you no good. Assuming what you see is true, you have no idea where that person has come from, the work they have put in to achieve what they have achieved or the struggle they have in life. You have no idea where that person is in their journey of life so it's silly to compare your beginning to someone else's middle or end.

Focus on your own goals and your own life. Look in the mirror, that's your competition. But I get it; you've got Facebook and Instagram showing you all day long these beautiful people having an amazing life. Ignore it. Focus on your own shit. It's not real anyway. It's a tiny snapshot of 1% of their life. If someone has a million pounds in the bank, they have million-pound problems. Everyone's life is full of the same problems. We all have problems, rest assured. Concentrate on being the best YOU that you can be, in every area of your life that's important to you.

"Don't compare yourself with anyone in this world. If you do so, you are insulting yourself."

- **Bill Gates** -

17. PROBLEM SOLVING & TAKING ACTION

"Set your goals. Dream BIGGER. Take action."

- Gav Gillibrand -

You've got the best intentions. You know what to do and why you want to do it. You've got your nutrition plan sorted, and your programme at the ready. But what are you going to do when it all goes wrong? Because it probably will at some point. There's no escaping that. Life sometimes gets in the way and ruins even the best of plans. You need to be prepared. Expect the unexpected and have a contingency plan in place. Accept that something may happen in life when you can't prepare the best food or get to the gym. By being more aware that something like this may happen, you can recognize in advance or sometimes avoid it. If you can't avoid it, you can at least deal with it, forget it, and move forward.

Here's an example of what I mean: Your child gets sick in the night, you're up twice dealing with that and you wake up exhausted. Your planned early gym session may seem even more unappealing now. You've got two choices. Go anyway and accept that you're tired (you might surprise yourself and still have a great workout). Or you can just skip it. That doesn't make you a bad person. It's your choice and you're tired, so the temptation to stay in bed an extra hour, especially when it's cold and dark outside, is way more attractive than getting your sleep deprived carcass to the gym or going outside for a run. I understand that, and I'd be a liar if I didn't say it happened to me. It has on numerous occasions. If you decide to go work out anyway, full power to you and well done.

If you decide to stay in bed, here's what you don't do. Don't get up and moan about it, choose a crappy breakfast and leave your packed lunch at home to spite yourself. Woe is me. You have missed one session. In the grand scheme of things, it won't matter one little bit. It won't derail your progress. What will derail your progress is you making poor choices with your diet because you're annoyed at what happened. If you've got kids this, or something like this, will happen. Accept it and move past it. There's always time to add an extra session in at some point.

You go to an event, a dinner party, or a work meal. You're on a calorie-controlled eating plan. You know there will be canapés and champagne on arrival. If you eat before you go, the chances of you going hog wild is seriously reduced. Not eliminated entirely but reduced. Go hungry to the event, have one or two glasses of champagne, and it's sayonara. Game over. Again, you have two choices. You've eaten 12 canapés and drunk three glasses of champagne, and a gin & tonic slipped in there somehow. You can limit the damage by stopping there, or you can go ballistic and get home at 3am. The choice is yours.

Perhaps you've got some big goals. They're ambitious, but now it's your time. You're determined to do it this time. You're finally going to stick to the plan. Enough is enough. The time is now. You plan to go the gym five times a week. That's great if you can stick to it but you've not gone once in the last five years. Going from nothing to 20 times in a month is a plan destined to failure for most people. Week one, you hit the goal. Week two, you've dropped to three times per week. Week three, you only go once, and week four, well the less we talk about week four the better.

Setting a goal to go twice a week for the next six weeks is attainable and achievable. If you go twelve times in six weeks, you gain momentum. You experience all the positive benefits. You start to feel good about yourself, and you lose a little weight. Your courage grows. Confidence soars and you can commit to a third session. You start to realize that you've always had time to exercise, you just didn't see the benefit or make it a priority. Make a plan that is achievable, even if it seems too easy in the beginning. Make a plan that allows a gym session to be missed. Make a plan that takes into consideration family, work, and life commitments. That's your plan. That's your life.

Taking Action

What needs to happen for your journey to be a success? We know that you're going to have to start exercising if you're not already, and maybe do a little more if you're already doing something. We know that you should address your sleep, cut down or cut out your alcohol, and increase the amount of water you drink, but above all, you absolutely must track your calories.

Let's say you're the owner of a bank. At the end of the year, you ask the bank manager, "did we make any money?". The manager says, "Well, I think we did. We took a lot of money in, and a lot of money went out, but I don't really know". It's a stupid scenario that would never take place. A bank would know every penny that was exchanged because it's recorded. It's the same with your diet and weight loss results. I'm not saying you must record everything with exact precision all the time, but if fat loss is a goal, recording and tracking calories is the activity I suggest you spend the most time on. MyFitnessPal, as I've mentioned before, is easy to use and it's effective. Maybe a little tedious at times, but it's not half as tedious and tiresome as carrying an extra 40lbs around with you all day long. Fat loss occurs when you're in a deficit. This means you're burning more calories than you consume.

I often get asked, "What's the best exercise to do to lose fat?" I respond, "a calorie deficit". If you jogged/walked for one hour at a very leisurely pace of 4mph the average person would burn 400 calories. Or you could decrease your calories by 400 by simply missing a few snacks. It's a lot easier to make dietary changes than it is to exercise for an hour for most people. The best exercise for fat loss is learning to put your fork down.

18. MYTHS & OBJECTIONS

"Myths that are believed in tend to become true"

- George Orwell -

The fitness industry is a funny business. It's probably one of the most misunderstood industries out there. Let's face it, if everyone knew what to do, they'd all have the body of their dreams, endless energy, and gaining weight just wouldn't be a thing; but we know that's not the case. I hear so many myths being bandied around from clients, the media, and indeed other fitness professionals. It must be very confusing when even the "people in the know" are leading the unsuspecting individual down the wrong path.

The media and celebrities must take their share of the blame. They constantly perpetuate and aggravate the situation by promoting products that very often don't work, with an aim of selling magazines first, and perhaps helping you second. It's frustrating to constantly hear ideas and philosophies that don't work and, in some cases, can be dangerous, that are often just total lies and bullshit. In a way, it's kept me busy over the last 20 years because if you all knew the truth, you wouldn't need a coach like me, so for that I'm grateful.

I could write a book just on the myths but in the meantime, here are three of the most common myths I've heard over the years.

Eating Too Many Carbs Makes You Fat

Many people believe that eating too many carbs is the reason they have excess body fat to lose; and that cutting or reducing this much-maligned macronutrient from the diet is the answer to their prayers. It's not and you don't need to do that. Put your hand up if you've ever said to yourself, "I'm cutting carbs as I need to lose fat". My hand went up, and I'm sure yours did too. It's not hard to see why. There are many diets available to the general public, lots of philosophies on how to lose weight, and yet obesity levels continue to rise every year.

It's clear to me that common dieting ideas about eating carbs need to improve. What you need to realise is that it's not too many carbs making you fat; it's too many calories. It doesn't matter where those calories come from. If you eat more calories than you burn, you're in a calorie-surplus, and you'll gain weight. If you eat fewer calories than you need, you're in a calorie-deficit, and you'll lose weight. It doesn't matter where the calories come from. Carbs are not your enemy. Too many calories are your enemy. If used correctly, carbs can be highly effective in your weight loss goals. More importantly, they taste great, and give you a warm, gooey feeling inside; or is that just me?

Take home point: Calorie reduction is required for you to lose weight. That reduction can come from carbs, but it's not necessary. The calorie reduction can come from any macronutrient.

Eating Too Many Eggs Gives You High Cholesterol and Heart Disease

This is a true story from a client of mine called Jack.

"I've started really well today. Got my protein in. Had one egg and half an avocado for breakfast, just like you said on the diet sheet you sent me". Jack smiled at me. Confident he's nailed breakfast and started his week strong.

"That's a great effort, but I'm curious as to why you only had one egg. One egg will give you about 7g of protein. I think you'd be better off with three eggs. You should try to aim for about 20g of protein minimum per sitting if you can".

"I'm worried about the cholesterol in eggs", he said. "Last time I was at the doctor's he talked about only eating three eggs per week, as they're high in cholesterol. My mum has high cholesterol, and he said high cholesterol is hereditary. He's got her on statins and if I keep eating three eggs per week, I might have to go on them myself".

Talk about the blind leading the blind. I'll be honest, if I had a pound for every time I heard a similar story about eggs and cholesterol, I'd have about 27 quid by now. Okay, I'm joking, of course, but it's a very common assumption that I hear often. It makes sense, doesn't it? Eggs do contain cholesterol; in fact, the average egg contains about 200 milligrams of cholesterol. The current guidelines suggest we only consume 300 mg of 'bad' cholesterol per day. The media often tells us that by eating eggs, our cholesterol will rise. High cholesterol is responsible for heart disease, isn't it?

You don't get high cholesterol from eating foods with cholesterol in, I explained. "The cholesterol you eat has a minimal effect on your blood levels of cholesterol. If you eat less cholesterol, your liver will simply produce more. If you eat more in your diet, the liver will make less".

Cholesterol is an essential molecule imperative to our very existence. Without it there would be no human life. It's a major structural molecule in the body. Cholesterol's negative reputation is largely unfounded. It's been unfairly demonized over the last few decades. Cholesterol is found in every single cell of your body. It's primarily produced in the liver and is a basic raw material that we need for many functions in the body. Your body needs adequate amounts to make Vitamin D and sex hormones, such as estrogen, progesterone, and the all-important testosterone. Alongside hormones it also makes the bile acids needed for digestion. We need cholesterol to create brain cells and some studies show that lowering cholesterol too much using statins can cause depression, aggressive behaviour, and cerebral hemorrhages. Yes, statins do exactly what they're meant to - lower cholesterol. But at what expense? Statins: the 30 billion dollar a year industry. That's another topic for another time perhaps.

We need cholesterol for memory. Too little cholesterol in the cell membranes and nerve transmission can be affected. This means you get a type of amnesia. It's also an important piece of the puzzle when fighting infections. It helps neutralize toxins produced by bacteria in the gut when the immune system is weakened. I could go on all day talking about why we need cholesterol and that for most people eating eggs every day is not a problem, but I won't. I'm simply going to ask you to do your own research. The best advice I can give you is to check out the book, *"The Great*

Cholesterol Myth", by Johnny Bowden.

Eating Fat Makes You Fat

This is a fictitious story from "David" who doesn't exist other than to serve the purpose of illustrating my point here.

David is strolling through the supermarket with a shopping bag in hand. He'd Googled a low-fat diet online and printed it off. It's low in calories, 1,200 calories per day with virtually zero fat. Perfect. He wanted to lose four stone. He was very stressed from a job he detested, which paid peanuts. His ex-girlfriend had recently dumped him, calling him fat. Bitch! He was fat though; he had to admit it to himself. 110kg, "fuck! I'm only 5' 6". He cursed himself and threw the scales back into his wardrobe that morning, vowing never to step on them again. He knew that was a lie of course, but for a second it almost sounded convincing.

David had been on every diet known to man and nothing seemed to work. Admittedly he'd given up after a few weeks when the results didn't come fast enough for him. That had always been the problem. Sticking to something and seeing it through. This time would be different. A 12-week, low-calorie, low-fat diet taken from the Internet is what he wanted and that's what he got himself.

Here's the thing. If David can stick to this diet for 12 weeks, he'll lose a tonne of weight, there's no doubt of that. Any diet of 1,200 calories will help most people lose weight, but it's the restricted calories, not the fact that it's low in fat, that leads to weight loss. The entire 1,200 calories could come from dietary fat and guess what? David would still lose weight, fast. The mix of macros is largely irrelevant for fat loss.

If fat doesn't make us fat, why does the government tell us, in marketing and advertising we see every day, to eat a low-fat diet? As I mentioned before, 1g protein and carbohydrate contain 4kcals but fat contains 9kcals per gram. It's over double the calories of the other two macronutrients. By reducing fat in the diet, calories can be slashed, taking someone into a calorie-deficit quickly. Calling an important macronutrient, the same word as a layer of blubber on our bodies was a mistake. "Eat fat to make you fat". It sounds right, like it should be true. That's part of the confusion. When you put weight on, you don't get fat, you simply have increased your store of adipose tissue. "Low fat" is a marketing buzzword; it sells products.

What you must understand is that food manufacturers are making products for you to buy, to make a profit; not for your health. If they can get away with plastering low fat on their product, it's been proven to sell more. Cereal is low fat, but it's high in sugar. A can of Coke contains no fat, but a lot of sugar. Eating fat does not make you fat. Eating too many calories, regardless of the source, will hasten fat storage.

A Word of Caution

Be careful where you get your advice. Stick to real science. Ignore the big dude in the gym. He may be knowledgeable, but he may not be. Just because someone is in shape, doesn't mean he or she is an expert or qualified to give real advice. Instagram is littered with thousands of "models" in amazing shape. Some give great advice, some give terrible advice and get the unsuspecting to buy products in the hope they will make you look like them. I fell victim to this when I was 17 years old. A big muscular guy at the gym told me to try these drugs. I looked up to him. I wanted to be like him.

"No harmful side effects, mate, you'll grow like a weed". It turns out he sold me fake drugs, which could have caused huge problems. He was right though. I grew. Specifically, my face, and my nipples looked like I was lactating. I looked like a bloated water buffalo. It was not a good look. Thanks for nothing mate.

Objections

I know what you might be thinking. "I'm different. No one has the same stress I do, no one understands what I'm going through". You know what? You're right. No one can understand what you're going through. No one has the exact same problems, issues, or life as you. However, most people's lives are equally time consuming and stressful, so please don't think you're any different from anyone else. You just think you are and there lies the problem - the story you're telling yourself. "But Gav, it's okay for you to tell me how to get into shape, but I don't have the time to even think of getting to the gym". Ahh, there you go again. Are you trying to tell me that everyone that is super busy, travels a lot, has kids, is tired; can't take care of themselves? Is that what you're trying to tell me? Not one person that has that going on is in shape? No, of course you're not because you know it's just not true. That doesn't mean it's easy of course. It's going to take some real hard work to break the cycle you're in. Everything worthwhile is hard work. It's a cliché but it's true.

All clichés aside, stopping believing in the stories you keep telling yourself could be the hardest job you have. If you still believe these bullshit stories, there isn't much more I can do to help you. Revisit the blue and red pill metaphor again. You have two choices. Stay where you are and blame external circumstances or get to work despite all the perceived obstacles. Ask yourself: do you want to be a victim? Or do you want to be a person that overcomes everything life throws at you? Do you want to be around to see your kids get married and have kids of their own? Or do you want to be the fat dad on the sofa, too tired and exhausted to kick a ball with your son? Do you want to be the best role model for your kids? Or do you want them to copy you and potentially promote their own teenage obesity and early death?

Sounds harsh, doesn't it? It is harsh, but it's also the stark reality. I think we all know what you really want, don't we? It's up to you though. Hard work or stay the same and get progressively worse. Truth is; there's no staying the same, you're either getting better or you're getting worse. In this case, you're choosing to either live your best life, or die.

19. YOU ARE THE AUTHOR OF YOUR OWN BOOK

"The best time to plant a tree was 20 years ago. The second-best time is now"

- Chinese Proverb -

Forget what you didn't do in the last six months, the last year, or even the last 10 years. Focus on what you can do in the next six months ahead of you. You can change a few key habits and make radical changes in your health & fitness, if you want to. All it takes is a decision right now; this very second, in a heart beat. A decision to just do it. You're the star of your own movie. You get to choose the cast, write the script, and direct the whole show.

You're The Author of Your Own Book

That book is called your life. Don't like any aspect of what you're creating? Change it. You have the power to do just that. If you've messed up in any area of your life until now it's time to take ownership of that mess and realise that you have no one to blame but you. Not your parents, your childhood, or your upbringing. Not your environment, your friends, or any other shitty circumstance. Sure, they contributed to who you are, but the buck ultimately stops with you. The moment you realise that, and take full responsibility for what you have and don't have, the better. The truth hurts, my friend. Once again, you have two choices. You can ignore it and hope how you feel will go away. You can hope that the weight you want to lose will miraculously drop off and life will improve. That's an option. Or you can take control and say enough is enough.

Before I wrap this up, I'd like to leave you with one last testimonial, hot off the press. This literally came in as I was putting the finishing touches on this book.

"I can't thank you enough for what you have helped me achieve. To be honest, I was seriously worried at the start of this programme because I had just invested in a fitness coach from the other side of the world that I had been talking to for just 20 minutes! I had nothing to worry about because that first call showed me that you meant business.

Fast forward to now, I've lost 14.5kg/32lbs in 12 weeks on your programme and my strength has gone up. I didn't see this coming mate. I still can't comprehend how easy it was to lose weight on your 12-week programme. I had a picture in mind at the very start of the programme of drinking meal replacement shakes and having to starve myself all day. How wrong I was. The flexibility of what you can eat in this programme makes it very easy and the best part is that it is a lifestyle that I can now continue on and maintain with ease, thanks to your coaching.

I will be passing your details onto anyone that has a goal of losing weight or even just improving their health overall. I hope you continue to have great success with future clients. Thanks again mate! Keep in touch and all the best in 2019"

Jason (NSW, Australia)

20. CONCLUSION & NEXT STEPS

"Finally, in conclusion, let me say just this"

- Peter Sellers -

Conclusion

If you've got this far and you're reading this now, I want to do two things. I'd like to thank you first for taking the time out of your busy life and reading this. Your time is precious, and you've spent at least a few hours getting to this point in the book. Secondly, I'd like to congratulate you. Well done for deciding to take control of your health, fitness and ultimately your life. My system, The "GHG" Method is quite simple in its approach. I won't sugar coat it. I will tell you like it is, but I like to do this with a sense of humour. If this book has been informative and made you chuckle, then I'm happy. If this book has been transformative then I'm over the bloody moon. Job done.

As I mentioned before, achieving results that last is really like baking a cake. You follow a recipe that's been proven to work. You don't deviate from the recipe too much or you won't get the desired outcome – an awesome cake. The fact that I'm comparing your health and your life to a cake is amusing to me. The irony is not lost. Combining the elements of nutrition, exercise and a bulletproof mindset is your ticket to success, and I wish you all the best in your endeavours moving forward.

Your Next Step

You still here? Great. If you are struggling with your weight, fitness, or any aspect of your health, I'd like to help you. To be honest, if you followed all the steps in this book, you wouldn't need anything else, but I understand that many of you may want more. My flagship-coaching programme is designed for men that are committed to losing 20lbs or more in 12 weeks or less. I take on new clients every month. If you'd like to apply for one of those spots, here's what you need to do:

Go to **www.gavgillibrand.com/apply** and book a call with me. After you book the call, it will automatically take you to a short form to fill in, which really helps me before we speak. We will get on the phone for about 30-45 minutes and take a really good look at where you are, what you want to achieve, and how we are going to get there. We will put a plan in place and work together towards achieving your goal. I look forward to working with you soon.

Gav Gillibrand

PS. The blue pill or the red pill. What's it gonna be?

ABOUT THE AUTHOR

Gav Gillibrand is a Fitness and Nutrition Expert who specialises in helping busy, executive men be great role models for their kids and leaders for their families, as well as in business. From a T.V appearance on "Blind Date" in 1993 to a distinguished career as a male revue artist AKA a male stripper, travelling all over the UK & Europe, Gav went on to become one of the UK's most successful personal trainers & online coaches having helped 100s of clients in the last 10 years to weight loss success. He's written articles for Men's Health, Hello! & OK! magazine and many more.

You can connect with Gav at the following places:

Website: **www.gavgillibrand.com**

LinkedIn: **https://www.linkedin.com/in/gav-gillibrand**

Facebook: **https://www.facebook.com/gavin.gillibrand**

Instagram: **https://www.instagram.com/gav.gillibrand**

Podcast: "The Health, Fitness & Lifestyle Show". To subscribe, go to **https://apple.co/2SZegZY** and if you feel the love, please leave a rating and a review. Many thanks.

Printed by Amazon Italia Logistica S.r.l.
Torrazza Piemonte (TO), Italy